HOSPITALS, PATERNALISM, AND THE ROLE OF THE NURSE

Jo Ann Ashley

TEACHERS COLLEGE PRESS
Teachers College, Columbia University
New York, New York

A Nursing Education Monograph

RT
79
. A83

3/62 Rainbow 10.35

Fourth Printing, 1979

85019

Library of Congress Cataloging in Publication Data

Ashley, Jo Ann
    Hospitals, paternalism, and the role of the nurse.
    (Nursing education monographs)
    Bibliography: p.
    1. Nursing schools—United States—History.
2. Sex discrimination against women—United States.
3. Hospitals—Sociological aspects. I. Title.
II. Series.
RT79.A83   331.4'81'610730973   76-7908
ISBN 0-8077-2471-8
ISBN 0-8077-2470-X pbk.

Contents

Introduction

THE BOOK YOU ARE ABOUT TO READ could as well be titled "sexism is dangerous to your health." It has been said that power corrupts and absolute power corrupts absolutely. A corollary to this is that powerlessness corrupts, too, by undermining integrity and inhibiting human growth. In this book, Jo Ann Ashley gives her account of how many men in medicine, health care, and hospital administration have kept nurses powerless and inhibited the growth of nursing as a caring profession. What follows will ultimately be recognized as a landmark book, long overdue. It is a book for every nurse, every physician, every health care practitioner, and every citizen who cares about the quality of health care in this country.

Ashley documents how American hospitals were established by men to offer nursing care actually provided by women, women who worked essentially as indentured servants. The male physicians and hospital administrators were preoccupied, as Ashley details, with control over others, profits, and male privileges. The female nurses were committed to service, to health education, and to the welfare of students and patients—important functions often discouraged by medical men.

What I'd like to suggest here are some healthy actions to correct the sexism documented by Ashley, and its contemporary unhealthy consequences and manifestations. To do this, feminist education must, in my view, become central to nursing education, practice, and research. In the past, sexism has artificially limited and distorted the humanity of health care practitioners, and health care and hospitals have been influenced by military and religious orientations, both of which are characterized by patriarchy and authoritarianism. This combination has impeded any chances for internal reform. The Bible teachings I learned as a child admonished us to treat slaves kindly but did not challenge the inhumanity of slavery as an institution. This is the basic difference between reform designed to ameliorate symptoms of problems and radical approaches aimed at the basic causes of problems. Most nurses have worked diligently at reform, but feminists are inherently radical. That many nurses have come to view the problems in their profession with a feminist perspective should be considered a very healthy development.

In chapter six Ashley discusses the origins of the American Nurses' Association and the National League for Nursing. Their divide and conquer approach and its consequences had these two major nursing associations competing against each other for minimal professionalism in health care. The real power to change lies beyond nursing's historically tragic drama of dependence and the artifice of ladylike powerlessness. The inability and/or unwillingness of most nursing leaders to identify until recently with feminist imperatives and their potential for nurses is understandable but no longer acceptable. Nurses have dedicated fine lives to reform, to service, to the welfare of others and we can afford no more false modesty or accomodation to own own exploitation.

Nurses make up the second largest professional group of women in the country. Nursing is the largest occupation among health care practitioners. Nurses, by the strength of their numbers, could be a vanguard, making health care as much a fundamental right in our society as is a public school education.

The feminist-led women's health movement represents a radical critique of standard health care with both economic and cognitive dimensions. These feminists recognize that health care is a relational phenomenon between people and that thus existential insights are crucial to its proper functioning. These feminist perspectives offer a means of demystifying health care for all society—men, women, and children. Nurses are beginning to ask the same questions that the women's health movement asks: What constitutes health care? Who gets what and how much? At what cost and under whose control?

Some nurses are now designing models for what health care should be, and how much better it could be without the hierarchical relationships and competitiveness that dominate medicine now.

Nurses should call on their own leaders, and the American Medical Association, to support the equalization of both job opportunities and monetary rewards in health care occupations, so that both will no longer be dependent on the sex of the persons filling the jobs. To its credit, the American Nurses' Association did, in 1971, reverse its longstanding opposition to the Equal Rights Amendment and has since become an effective advocate for its ratification.

In early 1974 the National Joint Practice Commission of the A.N.A. and the A.M.A. did at least listen to a presentation of feminist perspectives on health care. The recommendations presented included a proposal that the National Joint Practice Commission initiate a movement toward establishing the legal complementarity of nurses and physicians. The predominant situation now is that nurses are, in effect, licensed to practice under the guidance of physicians, as a dependent profession. This interpretation of the licensing laws hampers the effectiveness of the nurse and ignores the reality of many practice settings. The commission was also asked to encourage other health occupations to end the consideration of gender in determining who does what in and out of hospitals. In addition, the commission was encouraged to recognize the purpose and concerns of the women's health and "nurse power" movements. Were the A.N.A. and the A.M.A. to back these recommendations solidly, health care delivery in this country would undoubtedly improve.

There are now two groups of activist nurses working toward some of these goals. The A.N.A. has set up its own Nurses Coalition for Action in Politics with headquarters in Washington, D.C. Nurses-NOW, a task force of the National Organization for Women, is establishing branches throughout the country. When these organizations are successful, perhaps the American public will no longer be "more easily excited by the notion of barefoot doctors in China than they are by what their own nurses could do with their shoes on," as Ashley ruefully observes in this book.

It is not that nurses have done so little in spite of institutionalized oppression, what surely must be recognized is that nurses have done a great deal. As we remove the impediments of "men's work/women's work" from job descriptions, and recognize the dehumanizing effects of other stereotyping categories such as age, race, and class, we can create humanistic institutions including health care delivery that will be based on self-respect and love of others. Feminist nurses invite and welcome other health care practitioners to create the kind of world where the power of love exceeds the love of power.

WILMA SCOTT HEIDE

Ms. Heide was trained as a nurse and is a former president of the National Organization for Women.

Author's Preface

THE STUDY OF NURSING'S DEVELOPMENT in the United States is a study of overwhelming obstacles and lack of progress, of discrimination and exploitation. An historical approach to the study of nursing, medicine, and hospitals can contribute to a better understanding of current problems in the American health care system. Recognizing the origins of these problems may eventually lead to their more equitable solution, one related to patient needs and professional nursing's participation in meeting these needs effectively. Public recognition of the difficulties encountered by the women, the nurses, who attempted to improve health care can add to an understanding of how paternalism has resulted in serious and systematic injustices against women that have been both morally indefensible and socially damaging.

Though people differ on the nature of the crisis, many agree that there is a national crisis in health care. With the dehumanization and depersonalization of hospital care a major concern of the public, the crisis is undoubtedly a human one. The nation might not be confronted with the crisis had a system of medical paternalism not been dominant for so long. The social conditions that influence disease and poor health—sanitation, nutrition, cultural attitudes about health, preventive medicine—have all been within women's sphere of professional interest and activity. If the efforts of nurses to rehumanize health care and to improve the quality of the care given hospitalized patients do not receive more attention and support, even a national health insurance program is unlikely to eliminate the crisis, or the waste, or the standards that reflect poor quality.

Public awareness of the restrictive influences that have

persistently hampered the usefulness of the largest group of practitioners in the health field, the nurses, is a necessary step in any effort to reform our hospital system. The oppression of women in the nation's hospitals has not been an historical accident or a necessity based on rational justification—either morally, socially, or economically. Women's servitude in American hospitals and the economic utility of young women in these institutions was an outgrowth of prejudice against the female sex. Mythical notions and accompanying social misconceptions about women supported their servitude, keeping nurses subservient to physicians and preventing the full development of their potential contributions in the field of health care.

This study is the first of its kind to explore apprenticeship and paternalism in the hospital setting from an historical point of view. Much more historical research is needed before a complete picture of developments and problems in health care can be accurately assessed. Specifically, there is a need to further explore the political, economic, and social forces in communities around the country that influenced the growth of both nursing and medicine during this century. The rigidities and inflexibilities of mythical conceptions about the roles of men and women in health care and the resulting responses of community members need examination also.

It is my hope that this study, which examines discriminatory attitudes toward women, can provide both nurses and the public with an explanation of why nurses have had so little influence on hospital management. Though largely unnoticed and unexamined, the systematic oppression of the nursing profession has had far-reaching effects on the quality and delivery of health care throughout the nation. It is hoped that this examination of the effects of male supremacy in the nation's hospitals might break down some of the barriers that prevent the provision of quality care through the unnecessary waste of women's talents. Providing more personalized and humanized care for patients requires that those who care for the sick, notably nurses and physicians, be viewed more realistically in human terms as well.

Acknowledgements

WHEN A MANUSCRIPT is based upon ideas that grew out of a doctoral dissertation, individuals too numerous to mention have participated in the process of completing the published version. Original research for this study is reported in my dissertation entitled "Hospital Sponsorship of Nursing Schools: The Influence of Apprenticeship and Paternalism on Nursing Education in America, 1893-1948," done at Teachers College, Columbia University. Since the original study was completed, it has undergone numerous revisions and the dissertation committee is not at all responsible for interpretations contained in the final version. However, I still wish to extend my sincere appreciation to Professors Mildred L. Montag and Frederick D. Kershner, Jr., who co-sponsored the original study.

Thanks are also due my colleagues and graduate students at Northern Illinois University and to my family who, often without knowing it, gave hidden support in moments of private uncertainty. I will perhaps be forever indebted to my editor, who approached this manuscript with an open mind and enthusiasm. Several other persons read the manuscript and I would like to thank the following for their especially useful comments: Teresa E. Christy, Louise Fitzpatrick, Margaret Newman, Phyllis Campbell, Cheryl Stetler, and Marie Kalson. Final acknowledgements are due the Department of Nursing Education at Teachers College, its chairman, Elizabeth M. Maloney, and to Professor Marie Seedor.

Having learned many lessons about revising a dissertation for publication, I, as author, stand alone in assuming responsibility for the limitations and imperfections of a work of this nature.

JO ANN ASHLEY

Hospitals, Paternalism,
and the Role of the Nurse

I

Hospitals
as Schools

HOSPITALS IN THIS country developed originally as a manifestation of a charitable instinct which motivated public-spirited individuals to provide care for the indigent sick who, at a time of illness and dependency, could not help themselves. Rather than looking solely to public agencies for providing for the sick poor, these private citizens set out to devise a means of helping poorer working-class citizens regain health and thus remain useful to themselves and the community; the almshouses that existed then housed the destitute and helpless, but a stigma was attached to these institutions—people entered them, not for care and treatment, but to receive food and shelter, or to die.

In or about 1750, Thomas Bond, a Philadelphia physician, conceived the idea of establishing an institution solely for the purpose of treatment and cure of the sick. Bond consulted with Benjamin Franklin, who wrote the petition for establishing the first American hospital, which was presented to the Pennsylvania Assembly in 1751. His petition proposed the founding of an institution "novel" to Americans. While commending Pennsylvania's already established system of poor relief, he suggested that something else was needed for those having homes but lacking the means to obtain nursing care and treatment when burdened with disease. In short, it was thought, this deserving part of the population needed as-

1

sistance to restore themselves to their roles as useful members of society. A distinction was made between the objectives of the hospital and those of the almshouse, which was seen as an unfit place to recover from illness.[1]

This first American hospital was then a semiprivate corporation supported by private subscriptions and paying patients. In its early years the Pennsylvania Hospital had only a meager income. Despite this, the institution accepted those totally unable to pay, but of necessity, one of the earliest sources of revenue came from patients who could and were required to pay for their care. Though an outgrowth of an honestly charitable impulse, the actual incorporation and operation of this hospital was influenced by no less of a business mind than that of Benjamin Franklin. This charitable motive, in combination with the work ethic, led to the idea of social economy, restoring the poor to social usefulness, and was an important factor influencing hospital development.

Sixty years after the establishment of Pennsylvania's first hospital, the Massachusetts General Hospital, the first in New England, was founded and, despite the lengthy time interval, its goals were strikingly similar. In 1810 two physicians, James Jackson and John C. Warren, circulated a letter to "wealthy and influential citizens" in and around Boston. They wrote that Massachusetts needed a hospital to give the poor a chance to obtain "kind and skillful" nursing care under the supervision of a physician. The poor, by their definition, were those "having good and industrious habits, who are affected with sickness . . . and who have not had time to prepare for this calamity."[2] Again, the aim was to provide nursing care to prevent poorer members of society from becoming dependent upon public charity during illness. Society would profit more if these people, through preventive measures, could somehow be kept out of the almshouse.

The attitudes expressed by Bond, Franklin, Jackson, and Warren in establishing these hospitals reflect the value placed on work in American society. Their proposals suggest that charity had taken on a new meaning in this country where individualist tendencies dominated social thinking.

The aim of these hospitals was to help people regain their productivity; not to support poverty and dependency, but to alleviate it through preventive measures where possible. In this respect, care was not unlike an investment: those persons who were employable and could earn an income once well again were considered better risks than less fortunate individuals not capable of supporting themselves.

And so, although they have been associated in the public mind with charitable activities, hospitals have never been charitable institutions in the strict sense of the word. Almshouses were a form of pure charitable activity, but hospitals were not. Both public hospitals (supported by city, state, or federal money) and private or proprietary hospitals (supported by private endowment, charitable gifts, or religious institutions), and even some hospitals established for purely commercial motives, have always accepted both paying and nonpaying patients. Public hospitals have, of course, taken in greater numbers of the poor who could not pay. Private hospitals have accepted them too, but have kept their numbers to a minimum. Despite the fact that hospitals have always sought and accepted paying patients, much effort has been devoted to maintaining their public image as "charitable" institutions. The hospital's reputation and its prestige has been of major concern to its management, which until recently, has managed to preserve a "charitable mystique."

The system of multiple bed wards and private or semi-private rooms grew out of early distinctions between paying and nonpaying patients—charitable and non-charitable cases. The economic status of patients still determines room assignments. As commercial nursing homes have replaced almshouses for the aged, commercial considerations have displaced charitable motives in hospitals over the years.

Hospital care is big business. From the first, physicians and other hospital managers have insisted that the larger society would not benefit from the services of hospitals so long as these institutions were associated with free care of the poor. Later, when advocating economic and administrative reform in the hospital system, they insisted that an essential condi-

tion in bringing about improvements was a strict separation
of hospitals from all political control. On the one hand, this
view was partly a continuing manifestation of faith in individual initiative whether in public or private undertakings.
On another, it was indicative of the physician's growing interest in hospitals as centers for practice that would provide both
professional and monetary rewards.

At the turn of the century, new hospitals were established around the country at a rate of two or three a week and
the question of who should control these institutions preoccupied most meetings of hospital superintendents at the time.
Physicians were responsible for the establishment of most new
hospitals, and many adamantly opposed either public hospitals or government interference with private ones. At a national convention of hospital managers held in 1902, a physician summarized his colleagues' attitude by issuing this
warning about public hospitals: "Such a hospital would be
filled with people for free treatment who are able to pay for
treatment. The burdens of the taxpayer would be made heav-
ier; the medical profession would be deprived of a large share
of its legitimate practice; and a system of pauperization would
be established among the people."[3] His conclusion, supported
by his fellows, was that the best interests of hospitals could
only be insured by non-partisan control since "politics and
medicine never were and never will be mixed successfully."[4]

To a degree, the problem was influenced by the physicians' realization that there was a good deal of money to be
made from the practice of medicine. They were particularly
interested in the hospital as a solid business enterprise. The
chief administrator of the New York Hospital, a privately endowed institution, advised his colleagues at their 1903 convention: "The question of the possibility of conducting the
affairs of a hospital on the principles of mercantile business is
an interesting one and one which may well engage the attention of hospital administrators."[5] As a result of this commercially oriented attitude, the cost of providing free care, which
reduced the income from paying patients, was of particular
concern.

In that same year, the tendency of physicians to think along business lines in their private practice was encouraged by an editorial from the *Journal of the American Medical Association:*

> a little more business, a little more medical statesmanship and a little more attention to the materialistic side would not be out of place, and ought not to detract from the scientific and educational, but rather add thereto.[6]

At this time, physicians were continually urged to view the practice of medicine as both a "business" and a "profession." This development had profound effects on hospitals. In the first place, the thinking of physicians was significant because many were hospital administrators and members of the Society of Hospital Superintendents (which became the American Hospital Association in 1908). In their executive positions, physicians determined hospital policies. Secondly, most physicians eventually came to use the hospital in some capacity, while at the same time they maintained their practices as independent entrepreneurs not responsible for the operation of these institutions.

The increasing interest of the medical profession in hospitals encouraged hospital authorities to view their problems from the standpoint of business efficiency rather than from a humanitarian one. One physician's comment that the hospital system had always been a humane concern but "today it's becoming an economic question" was typical.[7] With the increasing use of hospitals by paying patients and the growing interest of the medical profession in medicine as a business, economic considerations became predominant and have remained so throughout this century.

The successful efforts of private individuals to establish hospitals and a belief in the virtues of private enterprise led to public acceptance of the idea that private control of these institutions was preferable to government involvement. For years hospitals had avoided any great dependency on financial support from government agencies. Despite management's fears of the bureaucratic control that comes with government funds, even private hospitals eventually had to accept partial support from public money. By 1909, for example, public assistance for private hospitals was available in at least 35 states.[8] And by the time of the Depression, the number of hospitals accepting this support had greatly increased. Though many were strictly private operations, they were viewed as institutions providing an extension of the state's benefits and were not only given public funds, but were also eligible for various kinds of tax exemptions.

In one decade alone—1900 to 1910—1,651 new hospitals were established.[9] A high level of interest in hospitals as potentially lucrative businesses gave rise to this unprecedented rate of growth. The majority of these hospitals were private, and quite definitely profit-making, establishments operated by physicians: "One or two surgeons organize small hospitals, of twenty beds, more or less . . . as purely money-making ventures . . . [these private hospitals] find their climax in some of the cities on the Pacific coast, where they are run with the same competition as any business."[10] Physicians had learned to capitalize on the respect accorded them in large and small communities throughout the country.

Many of these small hospitals were specialty hospitals, which confined their services to care of specific conditions such as tuberculosis, mental illness, children's or women's diseases. They were not general hospitals. Since nursing was the main service provided by these hospitals, it was from the sale of nursing services that revenue was produced. As early as 1897, nursing associations were concerned about the large amounts of money these small and special hospitals made from the sale of nursing service to patients both inside and outside the hospital. Nurses were major "financial benefactors" contributing to the profits made in such business ventures since the hospital kept the income produced by private duty nursing. Without the income from selling the services of nurses, it is doubtful that so many small hospitals could have been established or have stayed in business. Medicine was scarcely developed to the point of having many services to offer, especially in the hospital wards, but nursing was.

The beliefs and values of early leaders shaped the development of hospitals. As Charles Phillips Emerson, a physician and author, wrote in 1911:

> In America there is not, and never has been, nearly so strong an association in the popular mind between poverty and hospitals. It has ... existed in the case of certain hospitals and of certain wards in other hospitals, but this association is not true of hospitals in general. ... In this country hospitals are recognized as institutions for the treatment of disease, and they are supposed to provide suitable accommodations for millionaire and pauper. There is growing belief that a hospital is, or should be, a better place for a sick man than his own home, however rich that home, and consequently private hospitals and endowed hospitals are preparing to accommodate an ever-increasing and ever more varied demand.[11]

The public, both the poor and the wealthy, did increasingly turn to hospitals for care when sick. The popularity of "trained nurses" and their use of aseptic techniques along with the growth of medical science were major factors making hospitals more safe for patients than care in the home. More modern equipment and techniques prompted both the public and physicians to use these institutions in greater numbers.

In addition to their economic interests and their strong support of private controls, one other means by which medicine set out to strengthen its power in the system was through the use of hospitals for teaching purposes. The close relationship between hospitals and medical education was not established until early in the twentieth century. Prior to that time American medical schools were largely commercial enterprises independent of both hospitals and universities; they were conducted as private businesses and were often quite profitable. As late as 1910, the vast majority of the country's medical schools were of this commercial type, a factor accounting for the extremely low standards in medical education.[12]

The educational function of hospitals had profound effects on these institutions originally designed to care for the sick. After 1890, most hospitals established schools for nurses on their own initiative while the medical profession had to wage quite a campaign to convince hospitals that their educational function should be extended to include medical students. Recognizing that nurses were getting a far better clinical experience than were many medical students at the time, physicians began a campaign to get their students an equal share of time at the patient's bedside. Leading medical educators began to see patients as the best medical "textbooks" for the study of disease. A hospital to study in was, for medical students, like having a good library.

Hospitals did not, at first, see any major advantages in establishing connections with medical schools—their aim was to care for the sick, not to educate doctors. This was the direct opposite of their attitude toward the training of nurses. Nursing care was the major product dispensed by hospitals and to have a school provided many advantages, chief among them an almost cost-free labor source.

Initially, hospital schools of nursing in the United States were influenced by the results of Florence Nightingale's system introduced into English hospitals. Prior to her time, hospitals there produced more diseases than they cured. She had recognized the useful application of scientific principles in eliminating filth, disease, and death during her experience in the Crimean War. As a reaction against the dispensing of nursing services by domestic servants and the deplorable conditions in hospitals she promoted a system of apprentice training for nurses to improve patient care. In her day, apprenticeship was an accepted avenue into all professions and her plan for educating nurses followed these traditional lines, but was in addition a sound arrangement that included independent administration and financing of the training schools. The Nightingale plan provided for instruction in scientific principles and practical experience for the mastery of skills. A contractual agreement between school and hospital ensured the use of teaching facilities.

The introduction of trained nurses brought about a revolution in the English hospital system. The resulting improvement in patient care sent the idea to America and apprenticeship training for nurses was introduced here. In 1873 three experimental schools were established—at Bellevue Hospital in New York, New Haven Hospital in Connecticut, and the Massachusetts General Hospital in Boston.

The hospital schools established in the United States, however, differed from the Nightingale schools in one very important respect: they were not endowed and thus had no independent financial backing. In the absence of public or private support, the schools from the time of their inception faced financial problems of major proportions. An agreement by the school to give nursing service for the hospitals providing clinical experience was the primary means of overcoming this difficulty. This type of apprenticeship arrangement was the factor prompting hospitals to establish schools on their own initiative. Having a school of nursing became accepted as the most popular and least expensive means of providing nursing care. The hospital was the master and the student nurse was the apprentice, with the latter giving free labor to the former in return for informal training in the traditional manner.

Medical education did not at first have the same attractive advantages to offer hospitals. Hospital administrators perhaps assumed that the critical eyes of young men would be more disruptive than the willing hands of young women. However, despite much debate over the issues and opposition from many hospitals, medical educators were determined in their efforts to use hospitals as teaching centers. The growth and development of medicine as a science, displeasure with commercial medical schools, and the need to raise professional standards made leading physicians acutely aware of the obsolete quality of education in the schools of the day. Scientific developments gave rise to an emphasis on the concept of laboratory teaching, leading to a widespread feeling that a hospital was the best possible laboratory for the study of disease. Systems of medical education in Europe, particularly the German system, were selected to provide models.

Medical internships required in most medical programs today are an outgrowth of the model commonly observed in Germany. There, medical educators established close relationships between universities and hospitals. The great teaching hospitals in Germany held much fascination for American medical men; they wanted their own medical schools established in hospitals and connected with a university.

Responding to a well-planned campaign to reform medical education, hospitals did not long resist the idea of making their facilities available to medical students. Following the popular acceptance of interns, many large hospitals were increasingly referred to as "educational" institutions said to have a major teaching responsibility in individual communities and in the nation as a whole. The hospital's assumption of a teaching function in medical education did bring about reforms and improvement in medical education. Commercial medical schools were driven out of business. The end of proprietary schools in America did not, however, end the proprietary spirit that continued to surround clinical teaching.

According to Abraham Flexner, who assembled the authoritative report on medical education for the American Medical Association published in 1910, the proprietary nature of clinical teaching loomed large as a problem in both hospitals and medicine. In a paper presented to members of the American Hospital Association, he explained:

> Men engage in the practice of medicine and endeavor to develop large and prosperous practices. One of the means to this worldly end is a hospital appointment. . . . It is no secret that the professorship of medicine or surgery in a University Medical School to which a salary of a few thousand dollars is attached may directly or indirectly earn for the incumbent anywhere from twenty to fifty thousand a year.[13]

So in a very brief period of time the medical profession had succeeded in establishing connections with both hospitals and universities. In less than a decade and a half, medical education was said to have been "revolutionized." With these connections and with some professors of medicine able to make such substantial sums as early as 1911, it is little wonder that medical education could accomplish reforms so rapidly.

Nursing education fared less well in its connections with hospitals. No success story such as the one above can be told about reforms in nursing schools. Training schools for nurses originated in general hospitals, in close proximity to medical practice in those institutions. The practical work experience of student nurses was identical to that obtained by interns in medical, surgical, gynecological, and obstetrical departments of hospitals. Student nurses served a period of time in each department of the hospital, learning while giving care to patients with all manner of illnesses.

But schools of nursing had no university connections and were located in small hospitals as well as in the large ones used for medical training. Thus, the training of nurse students was entirely dependent upon the kind and quality of medical services provided by the individual hospital and the amount of attention its administration gave to its apprentice nurses. More often than not, this training was cursory and inadequate. The hospital was mainly interested in the cheap labor provided by apprentice nurses—as late as the 1930s many hospitals employed no paid instructors and provided little formal instruction.

The medical profession's belief in the economic philosophy of individualism, and their persistent efforts to maintain laissez-faire approaches in medical and hospital care, provided economic, educational, and professional advantages to this group collectively and to individual members. The power and influence of the medical profession had pervasive effects on the hospital system. Organized medicine feared any changes that would even remotely resemble socialism; thus, most any attempt to bring about changes for the good of the public was opposed by the profession because it was associated with the "evils" of socialized medicine.

Medical interest in economics led to increased talk about hospitals as businesses, but in actual practice any improvements in administration along sound business lines were more fancied than real. In 1920 hospitals throughout the country were said to be generally "poorly organized and indifferently administered," a statement which came from C. G. Parnall, the medical superintendent and director of the University Hospital at the University of Michigan. He added that improvements were greatly "handicapped by the popular faith in the degree of doctor of medicine."[14] Certainly a large share of responsibility for defects in hospital management derived from the influence of physicians since they established and ran most hospitals—hospital administration as a profession did not emerge as an entity until 1925.

At the time, some members of the American Hospital Association were ready to admit that one causative factor giving rise to nonstandardization in the field of hospital service was the lack of government control, or indeed legislative regulations of any kind. At their 1920 convention, a few administrators expressed the belief that the day of operating in a mood of individualism had ended, that the time was ripe for more cooperative efforts in hospital organization and service.

In 1922, Winford H. Smith, a physician and the superintendent of The Johns Hopkins Hospital in Baltimore, called attention to the dangers of a lack of social planning. He noted that "there is a distinct opposition more or less active on the part of the medical profession to organized community activities which include the handling of community medical problems by organizations" other than physicians.[15] Later, in 1926, the A.H.A. president told member administrators that they could no longer ignore the essential role played by their institutions in the economic life of society. He advocated less isolation and more cooperation with other institutions in the community.

Though fully aware of the increasing problems growing out of their laissez-faire approach, and the philosophy of individualism that was the predominant influence on hospital growth and the delivery of health care, the industry's officials, both those practicing medicine and those in hospital administration, refused to take positive action to change attitudes or bring about constructive change. The thinking of many physicians is illustrated by the comments of William Allen Pusey, made while he was president of the American Medical Association. In his 1924 presidential address, Pusey said:

> The danger in this situation is that the necessity for social co-operation tends to break down individualism and to encourage the less vigorous to look to society to do for them what it would be good for them to do for themselves. . . . It is an unconscious endeavor to set aside the law of natural selection and to counteract Nature's cruel but salutary process of eliminating the unfit. So far as the present social endeavor can be successful, it will tend to foster . . . to borrow Faguet's striking phrase, . . . "The cult of incompetence." The tendency is to foster mediocrity at the expense of competence. . . . Medicine is, in fact, particularly exposed to the dangers of socialization. . . . There is an evident tendency now to appropriate medicine in the social movement; to make the treatment of the sick a function of society as a whole; to take it away from the individual's responsibilities and transfer it to the state; to turn it over to organized movements. If this movement should prevail to its logical limits, medicine would cease to be a liberal profession and would degenerate into a guild of dependent employees.[16]

Pusey's argument, expressed in a variety of ways, has been and still is the classical argument set forth in opposition to changing the system of private enterprise prevailing in health care.

There were those who protested against the predominant mood of opposition to change. David B. Skillman, a hospital trustee from Pennsylvania, was critical of the medical profession. Noting that medical men opposed public support and financing of health care out of fear of the "dangers of socialized medicine," he stated: "They strive to maintain the status quo in this changing world." He concluded that medical arguments lost their validity when they were "suspected of springing from self interest."[17]

Skillman was in favor of a reorganization of hospitals. His solution, though not an original one, was destined to meet with no real consideration. He thought hospitals should be organized like colleges, giving "doctors the same status in the hospital as the professors have in the college or university. Make the doctors the faculty of the hospital."[18] Skillman underestimated the extent to which physicians would cling to a system of private enterprise—a system that best served their interests.

Hospitals as a business continued to grow rapidly in the United States. By 1930, the nation's 7,000 hospitals represented a capital investment that exceeded three-billion dollars, an investment comparable to many important manufacturing industries. Despite this growth, the development of sound policies of business administration did not emerge. A major study in 1929, sponsored by the A.H.A.'s Committee on the Costs of Medical Care, asserted that:

> in contrast to what has happened in the business world, the evidence indicates that pressure to achieve the most efficient utilization of fixed assets has been more or less removed from the administration of hospital finances.
>
> Many hospital superintendents have taken no part in the financing or the construction of the plant and equipment which are under their control. Their administrative efficiency has generally been judged by their ability to balance cash budgets for operating costs, rather than by their capacity to plan construction or to utilize most appropriately the capital investment under their control.[19]

A nationally controlled hospital system did not become a reality in American society nor do we as yet have a national health policy. Fifty years ago the average American was probably not as aware of problems within health care as are citizens today. Even now, hospitals continue to operate as local and individual units, each planning activities separately with a noticeable lack of cooperation with neighboring institutions. Lack of planning is still a problem as evidenced by fragmentation in care and duplication of services without improving quality.

In 1948 President Truman requested that the Federal Security Agency "undertake a comprehensive study of the possibilities for raising health levels." The report he received expressed particular concern with the idea of social economy, which had prompted public-spirited individuals to establish hospitals in the first place. Of hospital ineffectiveness and its contribution to national health problems, the report said:

> For the most part, hospitals have been planned, constructed and operated without reference to the economic and efficient provision of the wide variety of services expected in modern institutions. They operate mostly as independent units, without reference to one another, without arrangements to provide their patients, through integration with other institutions, the services which they individually lack.[20]

This indictment of hospitals applied equally to both public and private institutions, leading to the conclusion that individualistic approaches and a lack of planning and cooperation existed as problems throughout the country. Government involvement to that date had only slight, if any, effect in modifying the actual operations of hospitals.

Although modern nursing was an outgrowth of scientific development, apprenticeship in the field was essentially a method of educating nurses while they carried on the nursing work of hospitals. In a very real sense, the problems surrounding nursing development were the same as those in hospitals. Growing side by side, the social and ideological forces serving to shape the formation of modern hospitals also served to shape the development of the nursing profession. Therefore, any understanding of nursing must be viewed in the context of hospital development and its influence on education and practice in those institutions and in communities around the country.

The educational function of the hospital was beset by the proprietary spirit in combination with economic motivations; the formal advent of medical education and control in hospitals was a factor only adding to the difficulties in improving nursing education. The popular assumption that hospital participation could only add to progress in medical education and thereby improve the quality of care provided in the wards did not hold true for nursing education and nursing care.

II

The Business
of Apprenticeship

HOSPITAL SCHOOLS OF NURSING have, for a hundred years, existed as social institutions in this country. All nurses are familiar with the operations of these institutions for the vast majority have graduated from one of them. Those nurses fortunate enough to have received their education in collegiate programs are also quite familiar with practices in hospital programs because collegiate education for nurses is not yet liberated from some of the psychological effects or the more practical problems inherited from the long years during which hospitals dominated this field of women's education.

Prior to 1965 organized nursing tolerated hospital schools and the public fully accepted them as the major means of educating nurses. The public, however, is largely unaware of the similarities between hospital apprenticeship training and paternalistic systems common to pre-industrial times—systems in which individuals of a superior nature looked out for those of an inferior nature, such as slaves, servants, women, and children. The public, furthermore, does not realize that for decades the nursing service available in almost all hospitals around the country was usually provided by partially trained, inexperienced, and unsupervised nurse students, not graduate, licensed nurses.

When the first American schools of nursing were established the family was the institutional model for the operation of hospitals. All policies and procedures formulated to guide management of the "household" were designed to look out for the overall interests of the institution. Preserving the institution's reputation, its production, its progress, welfare, and efficiency were utmost considerations in the minds of those who made management policy.

The role of women (nurses) was very early conceived as that of caring for the "hospital family." Their purpose was to provide efficient economical production in the form of patient care; they were to be loyal to the institution and devoted to preserving its reputation. Through service and self-sacrifice, they were to work continuously to keep the "family" happy. All the departments of the hospital—from wards and operating rooms to storerooms and kitchens—depended upon the continuous presence of nurses. For 24 hours a day, nurses were expected to be versatile in their skills, to demonstrate their ability to take care of whatever needs might arise, whether in the area of patient care, medical treatment, housekeeping, dispensing drugs, or supervising the diet and the kitchen. Like mothers in a household, nurses were responsible for meeting the needs of all members of the hospital family—from patients to physicians. Continuous responsibility for the care of those confined to hospital beds is still a unique function of the nursing profession.

In addition, women (nurses) were expected to look out for the needs of men (the physicians) in the hospital family who, for the most part, did not reside in the household, but were free to come and go. In the absence of men, women were expected to assume full responsibility for their decision-making functions by taking on the male role themselves. This decision-making role was, of course, relinquished upon the return of the men. Nurses were, and still are, constantly supportive of the institution, especially of its male members, and constantly busy.

Considered full members of the hospital family, physicians were not restricted to functioning within the institution. Though often absent, through their influence and domination they carried the authority of "master." Physicians, male administrators, and trustees of the hospital board formulated policies and made decisions regarding the type of discipline and order to be maintained by the nursing staff. The doctrines of discipline, obedience to authority, and male-dominated control greatly influenced the function of the hospital hierarchy.

Nurses, on the other hand, lived within the institution and were generally restricted to working within it as well. However, there were exceptions to this restriction. Very often, particularly around the turn of the century, economic expediency required that the services of women be sold on the outside, in private homes, with the financial return contributed to the upkeep of the hospital family. In short, women existed to serve the institution in all of its functions, including earning its livelihood. Their role was not a specialized one, but a versatile one. As generalists, nurses moved from department to department, from one area to another night and day, providing services wherever needed.

Sex-defined roles have always been, and still are, the most outstanding characteristic of the division of labor within hospitals. For the better part of the twentieth century, young women entering training programs voluntarily subjected themselves to a term of economic servitude in which they were used for the good of the hospital. Under the yoke of a paternalistic system, long hours of free labor were extracted from them with little concern given to their health or personal welfare.

Though at their inception training schools aimed at preparing women for a profession, this function changed. Before long, establishing schools became identified as a profitable activity on the part of the hospital. By 1900, prominent physicians and hospital administrators (often one and the same) linked nursing schools with good business practice. Associating nursing with "conserving economy" initiated the beginning of repressive efforts that ultimately impeded the movement of nurses toward professional development.

In the first three decades of their development as a separate profession, from 1873 to about 1900, nurses proved their usefulness. Their skills were widely respected and they could insist on some degree of independence. The aseptic techniques then used by nurses were considered an essential part of the surgical practices of the day and surgeons would no longer consider surgery without the aid of a trained nurse. These women realized the extent of the physician's dependence on them. In 1895, Mary Alice Snively, a nurse activist, told her colleagues that the reputations of physicians depended upon the quality of care given by nurses. As she noted:

> The young aspirant for fame in the region of gynaecology who longs to rank among the successful operators of the day, [will not] think of engaging a nurse who is not thoroughly posted as to what constitutes the modern idea of surgical cleanliness, and is not thoroughly conversant with the techniques employed in the various operations in the realm of pelvic surgery. Or what obstetrician, whose proud boast heretofore has been that he has never once in his practice been obliged to write as a cause of death "puerperal septicemia," will not prefer as his co-worker in the field a nurse who understands [preventive medicine].[1]

Thinking in terms of the effects of good nursing on improving patient care, Snively felt that the time was past when physicians would entrust their reputation to ignorant and untrained nurses. Others in the health field seemed to ignore what was best for patients and nurses and sought to take advantage of the free labor of student nurses. Realizing their dependence on nurses, both hospitals and physicians felt they had to begin controlling their nursing staff and its training program. Hospital schools of nursing became associated more with labor management than with professional activity and hospital administrators worked to suppress their nurses' recognition of the importance of their knowledge and skills.

The importance of training programs to the economy of hospitals was a topic widely discussed at the turn of the century. George H. M. Rowe, a physician speaking at a national

meeting of hospital superintendents held in 1902, noted that
the first schools had been

> a special corporation engrafted upon the hospital, having an
> organization of its own and doing the nursing work in the
> hospital under contract. The school was not an integral part
> of the hospital, and hence was never under the authority of
> the managers, beyond so much nursing work for so much pay.[2]

Rowe admitted that such an arrangement provided for
the perfecting of training methods in the early schools. He
felt, however, that this had been accomplished and the schools
should begin to serve the hospital of which they were part. In
his opinion, a school outside the control of the hospital superintendent could well create "a system illogical, unbusiness-
like, conducive to friction, shifting the various responsibilities, and subversive of the best discipline." It could even
cause "warfare" and "disruption" of the "hospital family."[3]
Rowe pleaded for the centralization of hospital management,
for an authoritarian organization. His pleas were heeded as
this structure characterized hospital administration from then
on.

Schools of nursing, from 1900 on, were absorbed by or
established for the hospitals of which they were a part. This
absorption, the refusal to permit the schools to remain outside
the control of hospital administrators, was destined to prevent
their development as independent educational enterprises.
Allowing the schools to remain free from management, so
they could concentrate on providing women with a sound
preparation in the physical and biological sciences, would
have modified the nurses' role in caring for the hospital family. The strict discipline and the incorporation of the schools
into the hospital business structure almost entirely negated
their educational function.

In 1906, a prominent hospital administrator wrote of
the nursing school and its dominant position in the hospital:

> That the training school has become an essential feature of
> the modern hospital cannot be questioned. To attempt to con-
> duct a hospital at the present day without it, would be like

attempting to conduct business on methods which prevailed two or three decades ago, the nursing of the patients is almost, if not quite, as important as their medical care.[4]

The system of private enterprise in the health field provided circumstances ideal to the creation of oppressive conditions for women. The rapid growth of hospitals in the early part of the century, and an increasing emphasis on their economic function, were destined to bring with them commercial activity harmful to progress in education. The trend toward establishing apprenticeship programs, not as independent educational enterprises, but as a source of subordinate labor managed by hospitals, is illustrated by the manner in which the growth of training programs paralleled that of hospitals.

In 1880, while nursing was a new and unestablished profession, there were 15 schools. In the next decade this number more than doubled, and by 1900 it had increased to 432. A phenomenal period of growth then occurred in the first decade of the twentieth century, so that by 1910 the United States Bureau of Education reported the existence of 1,129 training schools.[5] During the same period the number of hospitals increased in similar fashion. In one decade alone, 1900 to 1910, 1,651 new hospitals were established.[6] This was an era of unprecedented growth both for apprentice programs for women and for institutions caring for the sick.

Many of the hospitals were small, private "doctors" hospitals, which were financially remunerative to the physicians who operated them because of the free labor of student nurses. Reliable statistics for the year 1905 indicate that more than half of these private, profit-making hospitals had "schools" for women.[7] Though the "hospital" may have been limited to 40 beds, it established a so-called "school" for nurses in order to obtain nursing service at the least possible cost. Innocent girls, thinking they were getting special training, provided the best source possible.

The public accepted this practice of exploiting the labor of these young women while promising them an "education." Even the administrators of leading hospitals made little effort to keep their economic motivations a secret. Long hours of work, competitive wages to attract recruits, and the selling of student services for hospital income were features of most training programs in their years of greatest growth.

Hospitals usually paid a small wage to attract applicants to their apprenticeship programs. This became an issue that caused much controversy among hospital superintendents. Most of them were more concerned about the effect of monthly wages on the supply of students than in its effect on the kind of education their schools provided. The question, which preoccupied much of the 1904 national convention of hospital superintendents, was whether or not training, board, uniform, and diploma were sufficient compensation for apprentice nurses. Many administrators maintained that the student did not have the right to payment since the schooling was compensation enough for the services rendered and admitted that they paid students merely to attract them in large numbers.

The Johns Hopkins University Hospital in Baltimore, long one of the nation's more enlightened and foresighted medical institutions, was about the only school that looked at the problem from another point of view. Rather than paying their students, they used some of the income from nursing service for textbooks and scholarships, and for paying instructors. The administrator of the Hopkins thought that a salaried instructional staff was a better way to spend the money and pointed out to the 1904 convention that, with the notion of cheap labor discarded, the hospital had been able to attract a higher grade of student. His position was:

> that every school in the country would profit by doing away with the payment of salaries, provided it was not done simply as a measure of economy, but as a measure of improving the instruction given in the schools. In other words, make the training-school what it ought to be, a school, and not merely a device for securing something for nothing; that is to say, securing nursing without paying for it. If you want good nurs-

ing you must obtain for nurses the best kind of instruction,
and you cannot get that without paying for it.[8]

Despite the approach used at the Hopkins, the majority of the administrators of small hospitals still maintained
that they could not attract students to their schools without
offering wages. Their students were quite often young wom-
en from families with limited means and they needed the
money. The hospital training schools knew this and took advantage of the fact that their students, while interested in
earning their own livelihood in a respectable manner, could
not get into or afford a university education.

In the controversy between educational and economic
concerns, economics won out and the practice of giving a
small wage continued. As late as 1920 the *Journal of the American Medical Association* recommended that the best way to
attract student nurses to carry on the work of hospitals was by
giving them a meager wage and providing housing. No mention whatsoever was made about improving the learning opportunities in these institutions and few hospitals ever considered employing graduate nurses to staff their wards.

Despite the use of wages to attract applicants, hospital
administrators occasionally found themselves faced with a demand for student nurses that exceeded the supply. In 1908,
the American Hospital Association began its organized effort
to solve the problems of the apprenticeship programs on a
nationwide basis. Earlier that year, the *National Hospital
Record,* official organ of the A.H.A. at the time, printed an
editorial commenting on the diversity of opinion surrounding the issue of the proper training of nurses. The editor
wrote: "There is only one organization in existence in America that seems fitted to broadly, impartially and effectively
deal with this subject . . . the American Hospital Association."
This opinion was significant because it ignored the possibility that either of the two nursing associations which had been
formed before the turn of the century should have an impact
on the direction to be taken by nursing education. The edi-

torial concluded that the hospital association could "bring to bear on the subject the layman's view, the nurse's view, the physician's view. . . . They can look at the question from a business standpoint as well as get the professional view."[9] What the writer did not consider was what would happen to the educational and professional aspirations of nurses when confronted with an organization controlled by management.

At its 1908 convention, the American Hospital Association did consider aspects of apprenticeship programs and set forth some minimum standards, which were really only recommendations for hospitals "to consider and adopt if they saw fit." Richard Olding Beard of Minneapolis, one of the few physicians who championed professional education for nurses, raised an isolated voice in questioning the actions of the association on the nursing situation. He criticized the predominant influence of physicians' private interests and emphasized that the problems should be looked at from an educational rather than a financial perspective. Beard said that "the sooner we deal with the question from the standpoint of what is fit for the nurse and get away from the question of what the hospital needs, I believe it will be the better for both."[10]

Another editorial comment in the *National Hospital Record* aptly represents the view held by hospital management. Indicating that the main consideration of hospitals was to obey the laws of supply and demand, it said, "each institution has its own peculiar problems relating to the care of the sick and a plan that may be desirable and easily possible for one hospital to carry out might, if applied to an institution differently situated, prove a burden grievous to be borne."[11] It concluded that progress in nursing must remain slow.

Given the predominant influence of management on apprenticeship education, leaders in nursing had little control over standards in the schools. The schools were privately owned, and nursing education and nursing service became synonymous terms in American hospitals soon after the first schools had demonstrated their economic usefulness. A concern frequently expressed by nursing educators was how to educate the nurse and care for patients at the same time.

Used as a means of increasing revenue to the hospital, the selling of student nursing service in the care of private cases outside the hospital was a common practice even before 1900. Reminiscent of the Middle Ages when the unexpired serving time of the apprentice was regarded as an economic asset and sold by the master for a profit, the custom was negatively sanctioned by the absence of any legal controls or regulations over the apprenticeship system and the practice of nursing. Although the nursing associations passed resolutions against this practice, their leaders were convinced that nothing short of protective legislation would stop it: the public would have to realize that it suffered as much as did student nurses from this particular use of the apprentice's time. A nurse directing a training program that engaged in the practice stated at an 1896 meeting of her colleagues the reasons given for justification of this abuse.

> The arguments set forth by boards of managers in favor of the pupils being sent out to private duty are two, the increase of the school revenue and the value of such training. I see no way of answering the argument regarding the finances. If it is necessary for the school to earn a livelihood in that way, it must be endured with the best possible grace, and a constant effort must be made to reduce its disadvantages to a minimum.[12]

Members of the nurses' association opposed the practice because students missed their formal instruction while in private homes and because it was unjust and unfair to the public and to graduate nurses. Out of ignorance, many families paid for the services of fully trained nurses while they were actually employing young apprentices with little training or experience.

Remuneration was paid directly to the hospital for student services sold primarily to non-hospitalized patients. This form of exploitation was most frequently engaged in by small hospitals, which were highly dependent on the income thus generated. As the superintendent of a Minneapolis hospital told members of the American Hospital Association at their 1913 meeting, training schools were an excellent source of income for small hospitals. Critical of fellow members for not being more "businesslike," he urged them to manage their schools in the following manner:

> Of course, each pupil should be given a varied number of a varied kind of cases to nurse privately in the hospital, and this service should be charged for at a rate of not less than ten dollars per week; we make it a rule to charge fifteen. And I look forward to the day when, for the pupil's own benefit, it will be the rule of training schools that each pupil must have a few weeks of private home nursing before her training can be called finished. And of course the hospital should charge for this service. Properly managed, the training school of even a small hospital can contribute a good deal towards the support of the institution, without any abuse of the curriculum.[13]

Some physicians, along with organized nursing, spoke out openly against this use of students, because they felt it was a gross abuse of apprenticeship. They deplored the fact that hospitals solicited private cases for student nurses by public advertisement and condemned the practice as graft. Ten years before the Minneapolis meeting, a Chicago physician stated publicly that he felt such "nefarious intrigues" on the part of hospitals were hidden from "medical men of honor" who were associated with hospitals engaging in such exploitative ways of making money.[14]

Physicians from other parts of the country also spoke out against those who abused student services for their own gain. A physician from South Carolina urged his colleagues to expose and publicly denounce those working toward the "furtherance of hospital graft." He condemned the practice as one interfering with the teaching of nurses who held positions "only less responsible than those of the physicians themselves."[15]

Despite the controversy it aroused, the selling of student services was recommended in hospital literature as a legitimate means of bringing in added income to the hospital. Some defended this use of the apprentice's time on the grounds that it added to the experiences of students. One virtue prized was that the activity instilled in students a sense of "loyalty to the institution, and inspiration in its welfare." The practice eventually died out when the increasing use of hospitals caused the need for home care to decline.[16]

Although the relationship between women apprentices and the hospital was a contractual one, a legal vacuum surrounded the apprenticeship system. Practices relied upon custom rather than law. The women usually received a small wage, thus the relationship between apprentice and hospital was very similar to that of employer and employee. By the 1940s and 1950s, most hospitals had stopped making any sort of payment to apprentices. By then most student nurses paid hospitals for the opportunity of carrying on the work in these institutions while being trained more vicariously than formally.

Early contracts specified the length of the term of service and indicated the amount of money allowance. In addition, hospitals promised to provide room, board, and instruction. Applicants agreed to remain under the direction of the institution, to be subjected to the rules of the hospital and the discipline of the school. Officials claimed the right and had the power to discharge an apprentice at any time for reasons they judged sufficient. Obedience to authority was held sacred under all circumstances. Questioning the rules of the hospital or a physician's orders constituted "misconduct" and students were readily dismissed for doing so.

Once accepted, pupils were required to sign an agreement expressing, in the words of one, "their willingness to obey all rules, to be subordinate to authorities . . . and to conduct themselves as members of a noble profession." The money allowance, when given, was not to be viewed as a wage since the education received was "full equivalent for the pupil's services."[17] Specific stipulations varied from hospital to hospital and changed periodically in each as the term of service, wage, and other features were modified.

Most hospitals required a probationary or trial period averaging from one month to three in length prior to having women sign contracts. This was the initial stage of apprenticeship, during which candidates were observed for their general ability to complete the term of service, their physical strength and endurance, their adaptability to the work, and moral character.

The training-school experience was also full of token rewards for apprentices as they moved from frightened probationers to graduates whose moral character and "sense of duty" had received the training school's imprimatur. Dress, from stockings to caps, indicated how far along in training each nurse student had gone. Apprenticeship ended with an elaborate ceremony of caps and pins.

As an attempt to improve the training offered student nurses, organized nursing encouraged the use of the probationary period for straight course work. One of the first such courses in America was established at the Waltham Training School in Massachusetts in 1895. Six months in length, this "laboratory" course provided instruction in the domestic sciences, anatomy, physiology, hygiene, bacteriology, and medical chemistry. In addition, instruction was given in "district nursing" (care of infants, and convalescents), "surface nursing" (care of the body), and finally, personal improvement. The courses were all taught by paid nursing instructors.[18]

In an effort to test the value of such instruction, Mary Adelaide Nutting, a graduate of The Johns Hopkins Hospital Training School and then superintendent of nurses and principal of the school, opened the second preparatory course offered by an American hospital. Begun in September 1901, the purpose of the course was, in Nutting's words, to overcome the "universal custom prevalent in training-schools of mixing theory and practice indiscriminately together with little regard to methods, standards, or logical sequence of subjects and with a totally inadequate provision of time for study."[19]

Establishment of preparatory courses at the Waltham and the Johns Hopkins training schools were attempts to alter apprenticeship training by using a more academic approach in teaching basic sciences. In 1913, an official committee of nurses in the state of Wisconsin recommended that the probationary period be used to provide instruction for pupils before they actually cared for the sick. This period, they urged, should include instruction in bacteriology, hygiene, and the principles of nursing ethics "with special reference to the rules governing the school and the hospital."[20] Official committees in other states—notably Ohio, Connecticut, California—urged hospitals to provide a definite course of study during the probationary period.[21] But little was done on a national basis. Nothing like the Flexner report on medical education appeared to arouse public indignation about the poor training and low standards that prevailed in hospital nursing schools.

The main difference was, of course, that medical students were primarily men, and nursing students primarily women. Society valued supporting the one and gave little thought to supporting the other. Political, social, and educational factors prevented nurses' organizations from having any major effect on the apprenticeship system of education. Hospitals were in control, not organized nursing. It seemed that economic considerations alone were sufficient reason to keep women in a subservient position.

As late as 1933 the administrator of the Massachusetts General Hospital of Boston admitted that the monetary value of student nurse service in his hospital was the main reason for maintaining a school. Employing graduate nurses, he thought, would place too much of a burden on the hospital budget.[22] Young women in training were still serving to support both their own education and the hospital.

Hospitals until mid-century did not assume responsibility for supervision of quality control in nursing care. Prior to 1930 almost all of the "head" nurses on hospital wards were senior apprentices, which gave no credible assurance that competent nursing care was provided. Apprentices in training could not be expected to provide consistent quality in service without supervision. Having students function in leadership positions was justified by the hospital on the basis that it provided valuable "administrative" training for nurses.

Even as late as the 1960s, it was the usual practice that students be "in charge" of nearly all hospital wards during evenings and nights.

Questioning practices within hospitals by the public as consumers of health care services is a current phenomenon. For decades the average citizen did not know what went on in hospitals, but he had been persuaded to believe in the moral integrity of these institutions. Hospital representatives perpetuated myths about their good-will and good-works in the name of education, charity, and their publicly defined mission of doing all in their power to provide the best of care. In reality, power over women and the sick, prestige, and profits have preoccupied the minds of most hospital administrators.

With students powerless to bring about change, hospitals made little or no financial contribution to the betterment of their training departments until mid-century. The provision of physical facilities such as housing was most often considered ample. Few institutions went to the expense of hiring separate faculty. In most, the regular staff of head nurses, supervisors, dietitians, and physicians served in the capacity of teachers, both by example and by giving meager classroom instruction. Learning was primarily achieved by associating with individuals on the staff, which really constituted a process of education by informal socialization into the system.

As the survey *Nursing Schools Today and Tomorrow,* published in 1934, reported: "In 1932, 23% of the schools did not have even one full-time instructor, and only 25% had two or more." The level of educational preparation of employable instructors in the field was just as deplorable as the scantiness of supply. In the mid-thirties, just under 30 percent of the salaried teaching staff had not even finished high school; of those that had, more than half had no college education whatsoever. Only 20 percent of the total number of training-school staff members across the country "had as much as one full year of college."[23]

This tradition of uneducated teachers continued for as long as it did largely because of discrimination against women. Until recently there has been little public support for the education of women in nursing. The public's attitude toward health care and the training of nurses has been that of letting hospitals do as they please. The public has not been aware of the contributions women have made to the support of hospitals and to the delivery of health care. Physicians' reliance on nursing service has been a burden for the latter. Surviving with little public questioning, apprenticeship education did not give rise to rapid progress.

Nurses were expected to pay for their own education by subjecting themselves to up to three years of labor in institutions that gave few returns equal to the value of that labor. The fact that direct public or private expenditures for nursing education were almost nonexistent until mid-century only served to further oppress women and isolate them in a system that was more exploitative than educational.

With the public's attitude of ignoring the needs of nurses, the attitude of hospitals remained one of viewing the education of nurses as of peripheral importance to the institution. This attitude is illustrated by the comments made in 1929 by Robert E. Neff, a hospital administrator and later president of the American Hospital Association. Addressing a group of nurses on the subject "The Cost of Nursing Education to the Hospital," Neff said:

> The placing of nursing education as first consideration is not to be expected. The needs of the nursing service in the hospital, instead of how many students may be properly educated, seems to be the basis upon which we operate our training schools today. Hospitals are proud to mention the education of the nurse as one of its chief objects, but cannot contribute to the development of nursing education to the extent that other departments . . . suffer.[24]

Although hospitals were "proud" of their schools, they devalued nursing to the extent of using the income from the nursing service to develop other parts of the hospitals. Despite the title of his speech, Neff said, "The majority of general hospitals do profit financially by their training school relationships."[25]

Members of the American Hospital Association simply did not believe that patient care or the social and professional contributions of women could be enhanced by less-exploitative methods of educating nurses. Wanting to retain private ownership of schools and thoroughly committed to existing apprenticeship arrangements, the A.H.A. board of trustees had in 1925 expressed the collective views and position of that organization:

> We are thoroughly of the opinion that a nurse should have a fundamental education in the theory and practice of many essential subjects, but we do not believe that the value of the nursing profession may be enhanced by any system which places preliminary education, theoretical training, and specialized branches in a class above hospital schools.[26]

With the commercial mentality behind the maintenance of hospital schools, these institutions were major instruments for women's oppression both economically and professionally. The development of the nursing profession could not be achieved in an atmosphere where control over the nurse's education resided in the hands of those who wished to exploit her for her labor. Indeed, apprenticeship as a social phenomenon has often been used as a means of keeping oppressed groups in subordinate positions and even in the United States it served for a while as a "transition stage between servitude and freedom," for both slaves and indentured servants.[27]

Nurses have not escaped the psychological effects of the oppressive apprenticeship system. Convinced of their inferiority and of the need for their subordination to the medical profession, many nurses identified with the system that oppressed them and worked to support its continuing existence. Nurses learned to believe in the virtues of hospital training. Early conditioning within these institutions intensified the capacity of women to aid the cause of their oppressors.

Apprentice nurses were taught to be loyal to the hospital, to be obedient and docile, and to accept the poor conditions of work and the stringent discipline. Repressive educational practices instilled in them respect for authority and a spirit of unquestioning loyalty to "master" institutions and to physicians. Nurses were not educated in a manner that might have led them to question the moral or social implications of a system that impeded their professional development. By design, apprenticeship education does not provide a liberal and general education. It most often stifles intellectual growth and prepares workers only too willing to conform to prevailing customs, traditions, and efforts to maintain the status quo.

Although it did serve as a profitable business arrangement for the hospital industry, the apprenticeship system was wasteful, particularly of the labor of women. The complexity of expanding practice in nursing *now* requires additional years of formal education in colleges and universities. Many hospital graduates spend years in an effort to obtain appropriate preparation for changing fields of practice. Others, unable to obtain the necessary higher education, are forced into monotonous and routine hospital jobs where responsibility is great but morale and interest low. Large numbers of women leave the field out of frustration.

Physicians and hospital administrators, even some who are critical of our nation's health care institutions, still do not see much of a relationship between the quality of care received by patients and the education of the nurse. Some physicians still argue that hospital schools must be maintained. Although it is a crucial factor in quality care, the education of the women who give most of the care to patients most of the time has not yet received sufficient attention. The importance of quality nursing is frequently not even mentioned in discussions on health care. For the public to come to some understanding of the current "crisis" and defects in health care delivery systems, an understanding of the largest group of practitioners in the field is essential.

III

Students
or Laborers?

MANY PROBLEMS IN NURSING closely paralleled those encountered by other laboring groups in American society. Hospital management had grown accustomed to the exploitation of apprentice nurses as a labor force, and thus the long hours of work expected of them became a controversial issue. Though conditions varied from hospital to hospital, and were often considerably better in more reputable institutions, the financial considerations that dominated management thinking usually meant long hours and poor working conditions.

The long hours of labor concerned the nursing profession for decades. Though many innocent and subservient nurses were led to believe that working ten and twelve hours a day was their responsibility and necessary for the good of patients and hospitals, others were critical of this practice. Mary Adeliade Nutting, ever concerned about the health of students, was one of the first nurse leaders to openly condemn this practice. In 1896, during an address to the Society of Superintendents of Training Schools, Nutting spoke of the reason for the long hours:

> The explanation of the origin of the preposterously long hours of service . . . exists in the fact that, as a rule, provision had not been made for a sufficient number of pupil nurses. Such attempts at economy in hospital administration are unwise and cannot be too strongly condemned.[1]

Nutting went on to compare the hours of pupil nurses to those of laboring men:

There is no other work sufficiently like nursing to serve adequately for purpose of comparison, but to take the first that comes to mind it may be said that from 56 to 60 hours a week are generally considered fair working hours for the laboring men. I believe I am right in stating that few industries require their employees to work more than 10 hours daily and their Sundays are usually free. We cannot actually compare industries with training schools, nor wage-earners with pupils receiving their training in an educational institution, but we can state that a pupil in a training school may work harder to receive her training than a laboring man to support his wife and family, for here we find in one of the most difficult and responsible careers a woman can undertake, that her only method of receiving a certain kind of education is not to work 60 hours per week, but a number of hours varying from that number to 105.[2]

In Nutting's opinion, the long hours of ward duty placed pupils in a position of servitude. She condemned such practices as based on unjust, ignorant, and shortsighted policies. With other nursing leaders, Nutting was particualrly critical of the commonly held view that pupils could work from nine to thirteen hours a day and still be able to function in classes and lecture sessions in the evening. In 1897 only one school of nursing, The Johns Hopkins in Baltimore then headed by Nutting, operated on the basis of the eight-hour day. The practice did not take on nationally, mainly because hospitals considered student nurses their nursing staff more than their students. This practice of using apprenticed young women as the main nursing staff of the hospital continued to mid-century and beyond, and is one of the reasons why hospital costs were kept artificially low for decades, creating a problem our health care system still must deal with.

Nutting's condemnation of this misuse of nursing students had little effect. In the next decade, the issue of long hours became involved in other controversies: one over whether or not nurses should become part of the national labor movement, and the other over whether or not state legislatures should get involved in regulating apprenticeship training programs and staffing procedures within hospitals. The long hours of labor also hampered any significant progress toward making the training program a truly educational process: a shorter working day would have given some time for real course work by students.

The opposition kept getting the issue confused, as illustrated by an editorial printed in the *National Hospital Record* nearly ten years after Nutting condemned the long hours. The editor wrote that everyone connected with the hospital would certainly like a shorter day, from the superintendent to the "lowly intern." But the hospital, he declared, was not like a factory or a department store; the needs of patients could not be confined to an eight-hour day—a comment nurses would hardly have disagreed with, but he was missing the point. The editorial went on to say that:

> hospital life is full of emergencies, its needs can never all be catalogued, and any form of legislation that would hinder it in its lifesaving work would surely come sooner or later under the ban of public disapproval. How could such legislation be enforced even if it were secured?[3]

No one argued that the hospital should be closed down at six like a store or factory. The need for shorter hours was because the nursing staff was composed of young women who were supposed to be students and who should have been allowed time for course work. Furthermore, hospitals worked these students such long hours so they would not have to hire graduate nurses and pay their salaries.

In addition, the "lowly intern" and the licensed physician, who admittedly worked long hours too, received, or in the future expected to receive, compensation for their labor. Physicians at the time were beginning to realize that much money could be made in the practice of medicine, and they knew the direct relationship between the hours of labor and the amount of remuneration. The graduate nurse, on the other hand, was often fortunate to find even a poorly paid position in a home or in public service agencies, regardless of the number of hours she was willing to work.

This "ban of public disapproval" the editor referred to would surely have fallen on hospitals themselves had the public realized that during much of the day patients were cared for by unsupervised young women with only one or two years of training at most. Persisting in her efforts to bring public attention to bear on the situation, Nutting in 1918 wrote to Mrs. F. S. Meade, chairman of the State Council of National Defense in Massachusetts, encouraging her to give some thought to a study of working conditions in hospitals. Nutting told Meade:

> Such a condition of affairs in institutions devoted to the humane and merciful purpose of caring for the sick, is, it seems to me, open to the severest criticism, and I do not believe the good representatives of any city would wish, if they knew it, to allow such a state of affairs to exist. It seems to me shocking to have to describe a condition which I know exists in many of our institutions at a time when we are cheerfully creating laws to secure an eight-hour day for men in our great industries.[4]

The public was largely unaware of the controversy over who did what for how long in hospitals. A letter written in 1918 to Isabel Stewart, a staff member of the Division of Nursing Education at Teachers College in New York City, illustrates this. Not aware of any major effort on the part of the nursing profession or anyone else to improve conditions of work in hospital schools, W. A. Baker, a physician from Virginia, wrote to Stewart:

> I wish to call your attention to an abuse that should be corrected; it is the long hours of service required of pupil nurses.
> We have societies that look after dogs, horses, birds, and fishes, yet so far I have not heard of any society or individual coming to the aid of pupil nurses.[5]

Baker commented that "conscientious" physicians and graduate nurses were becoming more and more hesitant to recommend nursing as a field for young women to enter, and continued:

> Our government has regulated the hours of service for stalwart men to eight hours. I don't know of any railroad men or government service men who have as tiresome, nerve-racking work as the pupil nurse.
>
> I think it next to criminal to require a young girl to go at breakneck speed over hard floors for ten consecutive hours. . . . Then some training schools require twelve hours when on night duty for weeks. The idea of a special serving sixteen hours! Horror of horrors—Shades of the Spanish Inquisition![6]

Baker's letter is of particular interest for two reasons. First, even though he was a practicing physician, he was unaware that nursing or any other organized group had actively carried on campaigns to cut down on abuses in hospital schools. Secondly, Baker had two daughters who were determined to be nurses despite his opposition. His letter was prompted by his attempt to obtain information about schools that maintained good standards and humane working conditions. He had no desire to see his own offspring enter the kind of school with which he was familiar.

Baker's comments demonstrate the lack of collective action by those in the health field devoted to the solution of problems in the hospital on either the national or state level. Had there been any noticeable movement toward improvement, interested men like Baker would surely have known about it. Since Nutting, who then headed the Teachers College Nursing Division, had long been actively attempting to correct such abuses, she responded to Baker's letter. She pointed out that nurses for some time had tried to correct the adverse conditions of which he spoke. She noted that hospital managers and boards of trustees determined the hours of work and other practices in training schools and that the efforts of organized nursing had accomplished few improvements. As she suggested:

> No greater influence could be brought to bear upon this whole problem than that which could be exercised by the med-

ical profession, and consequently your letter brings me a sense of real satisfaction, for I believe it would be within the power of the medical men to bring us much nearer a solution of the whole question than we can hope to reach by our unaided efforts within any reasonable period.[7]

Following this correspondence with Nutting and Stewart, Baker set out to inform his colleagues of the need for a hospital reform effort. In September 1919, he presented a paper to his county medical society called "A Flagrant Injustice" in which he attacked "profiteering" and the resulting "destruction of the health and future usefulness of young womanhood."[8] Despite his personal interest in the situation, Baker did not exaggerate much; moreover, his interest had prompted him to do his own research on the subject.

Baker had reason to believe that many of his colleagues in the medical profession cared little or nothing about correcting conditions in hospitals. He had written an article for the *Journal of the American Medical Association,* but the editor had refused to publish it because he thought "there were a great many schools that treated the pupils with every consideration." Baker was more inclined to suspect that his article was "too vehement" or "the editor may have had some friends conducting so-called training schools that he did not wish to interfere with."[9]

At any rate, this physician did impress upon his local colleagues the importance of taking a stand and they unanimously passed a resolution condemning the custom in American hospitals of requiring excessively long hours of service. The resolution urged the Virginia legislature to enact laws banning this practice, but it was ignored.

The next year the National League of Nursing Education initiated a different type of campaign to improve conditions without the aid of laws. Their effort had some effect, for by 1923 several of the better schools in the country had achieved a 56-hour work-week for students. This was only a minute step forward, because the majority of schools still failed to "provide one day's rest in seven."[10] Moreover, the work-week in many schools did not include time spent in class

—this was additional time added to the schedule of the student. Hospitals assumed that students could learn nearly all the nursing they needed to know while actively engaged in the process of doing it.

The increasing interest of nurses in obtaining a shorter working day was in part an outgrowth of similar interests of the labor movement, but a shorter day was also considered desirable for the betterment of their education. Representatives of hospital management did not, however, view the idea of a shorter day as at all desirable. Some administrators openly expressed their resentment over the influence the labor movement was beginning to exert on hospitals, as evidenced by the number of editorials and conferences on the subject.

Hospitals in California became the first exception to the general rule that these institutions were exempt from legislative measures designed to curtail the hours of work of women employees. The inclusion of hospitals under the provisions of a law that regulated the hours women could work in the state of California created a nationwide controversy in the health field that lasted for more than a decade.

In 1911, the California legislature limited the number of hours women could work, but the law did not include the women employed by hospitals, who were almost entirely student nurses. For the next two years pressure mounted to include these young women under the protection of the law. As recalled by Mrs. Charles Farwell Edson, a member of the California Industrial Commission, at a convention of nurses held in 1915:

> I soon began to hear from people who had been in hospital wards, and from relatives of young women who were students. They did not understand why if there was an eight-hour law for women in California these young women did not have the privileges of such protection. Complaint after complaint came to the Los Angeles and San Francisco office. . . . Complaints so constantly coming in made us believe that an amendment to include student nurses would be a valuable thing.[11]

Mainly as a result of pressure by the labor movement in California, the state legislature passed a bill to protect student nurses under the provisions of the 1911 law. It was enacted in 1913, making it the first piece of labor legislation in the nation to include hospitals, and therefore student nurses, under its provisions. As reported to the National League of Nursing Education in the year of its passage:

> In California the Governor has signed a bill for the protection of the women which provides for an eight-hour day, and applies to pupil nurses in hospitals. It does more. It provides for a 48-hour week, and thus for the first time in history that class of working women known as pupil nurses will have one day off in the week.[12]

Despite this enthusiastic appraisal, many nurses objected to it because it classed them with labor as a trade. The bill's adoption led to the staffing pattern now used in all modern hospitals, that of three eight-hour shifts. The eight-hour day meant that hospitals had to employ half again as large a nursing staff to maintain the same number of women on duty at a time.

Hospital administrators vehemently opposed the bill. Not only did it necessitate increasing their nursing staff, it also limited their ability to use the student nurses as a source of revenue for the hospital. An incidental provision of the law made it illegal for hospitals to charge for the services of student nurses working on private cases. This meant the loss of a considerable amount of income, particularly for the small private hospitals. Two years later, when the state's hospitals were making a last attempt to change the law, the testimony given by a San Francisco Labor Council representative indicated just how much this could be:

> Investigations have shown that they [student nurses] are both underpaid and overworked. Undergraduate nurses received from $15 to $12.50 a month while the patients are charged $25 a week for their services and $7 to $10 for their board, giving the hospitals a profit of some $125 a month for each girl.[13]

The owners of proprietary hospitals, who most frequently took advantage of student nurses to produce extra income, were most vigorous in their opposition to it. As a nurse from Pasadena reported:

> We are told it has increased hospital rates, that it has or may jeopardize lives on the operating table, that patients have been rebuffed with allusions to the law, making the patients feel responsible for permitting an absurd measure to be passed, that doctors are displeased with the service. . . . A disposition to make the law appear vicious, and detrimental to the good of all concerned rather than to conform with it, or at least live up to the spirit of the law . . . has been noticeable. The greatest loss to the hospitals no doubt was the income from pupil nurses on special duty. Just how great this revenue was may be estimated when we have reason to believe that in some institutions 40 percent of the nurses were on special cases. Frequently probationers were assigned to special duty and some nurses have estimated that two-thirds of the time, while enrolled as student nurses, was given to special duty.[14]

Eventually the U. S. Supreme Court was brought into the controversy. Representatives of California hospitals took their case to the Court, claiming that the law was unconstitutional because it violated the student nurses' freedom of contract. The Court's opinion, written in 1915, which upheld the California statute, read in part:

> restriction as to the hours of employment of student nurses in hospitals is not an unconstitutional violation of the freedom of contract, as these persons, upon whom rests the burden of immediate attendance upon and nursing of patients in hospitals, are also pupils engaged in a course of study and the propriety of legislative protection of women undergoing such a discipline is not open to question.[15]

A significant aspect of the Supreme Court decision was its implication that student nurses were laboring women as well as students, a judgment that did not sit well with many nurses. They had, after all, been trying for years to have student nurses recognized as women training for a profession rather than as laborers. Unfortunately, these women were to a large extent ignoring reality. Hospitals exploited the labor of their apprentice nurses just as much as many other industrial organizations exploited the labor of their employees at the time. These nurses did have a point—being classified as labor would hardly aid their acquisition of professional status. But other attempts at obtaining legislation for nurses resulted in nothing: no legislatively decreed standards of training, and no mandatory registration of those who sought to call themselves nurses.

The real controversy was best summed up by Annie W. Goodrich, a widely respected nurse activist. As she said to her colleagues in the National League of Nursing Education in 1915:

> If our schools were really schools it would not be possible for them to be under any labor law. . . . The greatest indictment against hospitals and training schools was made when the labor organizations were obliged to put that eight-hour law into effect. I do not believe it would have gone into effect if the labor organization had not put it into effect.[16]

So the conflict over the California law was really part of the conflict about the training of a nurse. Were the diploma and cap awarded to the young women who completed nurse training to signify that they had acquired some substantial knowledge about the human body and diseases that might strike it? Or was it just to signify that they had emptied bedpans, rolled bandages, and made beds for two or three years? The number of hours of labor was incidental to the basic issue of what the function of the trained nurse was to be. None of the nurse leaders, whether or not they supported the California legislation and the coalition with labor it implied, would insist that a student nurse should quit in the middle of an operation, or leave a needy patient untended, just because her eight hours were up. The problem was that most student nurses were serving responsible functions in the hospitals to which they were apprenticed, but these same hospitals refused to grant these young women the status and dignity that their function should have received, and this was largely due to their sex.

California's new law did not apply to graduate nurses, who were still free to work any number of hours they wished, in either hospital service or private duty. As Mrs. Edson, of the California Industrial Commission and a stalwart advocate of the law, explained the year after its passage:

> Graduate nurses are still permitted to work as long as they choose, but we felt that it is unfair to the public to permit student nurses to be put on cases that require skilled attention and kept on them for weeks at a time at the rate charged for trained nurses. That frequently has been done to the detriment of the nurse and patient. Since patients dislike a frequent change of nurses, it becomes necessary for trained nurses to attend only serious cases, which is good for the enforcement of the eight-hour law, but which has excited the animosity of the commercial hospitals, which are forced to pay higher wages for skilled attention. But the public profits, if the hospitals do not, from this change.[17]

Though little affected by the law, graduate nurses in California did have understandable grounds on which to object to it. Not only did it imply that their training was laboring rather than professional preparation, the limitations it imposed on California hospitals did not substantially improve graduate nurses' chances for full employment. Rather than hiring, and paying, graduates to serve as their nursing staff, hospitals simply increased the number of women admitted to apprenticeship programs. This, of course, intensified unemployment problems as hospitals turned out more and more graduate nurses.

In 1914 the *Pacific Coast Journal of Nursing* reported a major oversupply of nurses. Graduates were "daily turned away from registries" because of a lack of sufficient jobs. Graduates were urged to come to California "as visitors only" and "not with the expectation of easily making a livelihood."[18] California could not absorb its own graduates let alone "floaters" who might drift to that state hoping to find employment. The very term "floater" was a word used frequently to describe graduate nurses in their search for employment—a graphic term depicting the manner in which nurses drifted from job to job, city to city, and, less frequently, from state to state. "Floaters" were criticized for their lack of roots and for their being transients, constantly on the move looking for jobs. These combined to make them less than desirable to hospital officials as possible employees.

The opposition to labor legislation put forth by nurses themselves was part of the difficulty faced by organized nursing in advocating change. Many nurses had resented the hardships of the long hours of work required of them during training, but apparently they seldom questioned the necessity of it. Such unquestioning subservience is bound to result from an apprenticeship system of training. When an occupation has little independent status itself, as has been the case with nursing for most of its history, practitioners would assume the status of the institution for which they were working, as subservient women have done for centuries. Any identification with labor would undermine this precarious sense of worth.

The efforts of organized nursing to improve working conditions and to lessen the exploitation of nurses were often misinterpreted by many nurses themselves, as the California law had been. They riled at being called "trade unionists," "class oriented," and "un-American," names thrown at nurses who supported laws to regulate their practice.[19] In addition, for nursing to be classified with labor as a trade provided another basis for those arguing against elevating educational standards. Laborers did not require a higher education, let alone professional preparation.

Many representatives of organized nursing in California were adamantly opposed to the law and had actively campaigned against its passage. Anna C. Jamme, who was active in the California State Nurses' Association and the major proponent of a nurse practice act for the state, was one of many opposed to the bill. Her opposition was not against the need for a shorter working day but because she had hoped the national nursing associations could solve the problem of long hours in a more "dignified manner."[20] Jamme revealed her concerns in a letter written in 1913 to Mary Adelaide Nutting at Teachers College, who felt quite differently about the matter. Nutting replied:

> I am really not a bit worried about the dignity of the profession of nursing, and I am sure that you will some day agree with me. It is entirely true, as your legislators state, that nurses everywhere are overworked and underpaid. Among those who believe in the true dignity of labor, we should rank high and not feel that anything but good can come of the efforts of labor organizations to help those who labor.[21]

In another letter to Jamme, Nutting stressed even more strongly her views on the matter of long hours and the efforts of labor organizations to improve conditions for workers in hospitals:

> I have always, as you know, been in favor of shorter hours for nurses. . . . I think that the hours of work now required of pupil nurses and graduate nurses in hospitals and out of them, are oppressive, a menace to the health of the workers and indirectly in certain ways, to the health and welfare of those for whom they care. I am solidly in favor of an eight-hour day and night, and if the philanthropists and others throughout our country are unwilling or unable to secure proper conditions of work for their pupils and other workers, among which I include young hospital interns, in my opinion it is time for labor to step in and control the matter. I see no real loss of dignity in so doing; yet I know how you all feel, that in some way the dignity of our profession will be impaired and the status of nursing lowered, and I wish it were possible to secure righteous conditions for our workers in other ways. Experience covering half a century and over, appears to show that this is difficult if not impossible of accomplishment.[22]

Other nurses in California supported the position taken by Nutting. Representing the viewpoints of many nurses in private practice, they were puzzled over the actions of the nursing leaders who opposed the bill because of labor involvement. A nurse from Los Angeles wrote to Nutting about the divided opinion on the matter:

Now, we have the curious spectacle of *all* hospital authorities, most training school superintendents, and the medical profession generally, all clamoring for the repeal of a law, the need of such law having been so clearly shown.

The attitude of those in charge of training schools is what puzzles graduate nurses. Why they did not at once start their eight-hour system—a system that ought to have been established in all training schools ere now—without exhibiting such bitter antagonism toward the law, is a matter for surprise. By it, as well as the many strange reasons given by hospitals to the newspapers, conveying false impressions to the public as to the meaning of the law. The many nurses who would gladly have voted for any reasonable amendment, have now lost all sympathy excepting for the student nurse and have decided to use all their influence against the repeal of the eight-hour law.[23]

California hospitals did comply with the law, but only reluctantly. In 1915, the year of the Supreme Court decision, H. T. Summersgill, a physician who was superintendent of the University of California Hospital and at the time president of the American Hospital Association, complained about the effects of the law to the association's membership.

Much has been said and written pro and con on the eight-hour law for nurses. The constitutionality of this law was passed on by the Supreme Court of the United States. . . . On its face it appears to be contrary to the principles of not only the American Constitution but to all principles of humanity. For we all recognize the impossibility of strictly limiting the hours of attendants, nurses and others engaged in taking care of the sick.[24]

Summersgill was trying to have it both ways—a nursing service as professionals and as laborers. On one hand, he wanted his nursing staff to be available at all hours to work as long as the situation demanded, which is an obligation imposed on professionals but not on laborers. On the other hand, he wanted his nursing service, of which much was required, to be composed purely of subservient young women who would never presume to question their superiors.

Even after the Supreme Court decision had gone against them, hospital owners in California continued to fight the restrictions of the law. They concentrated their efforts on an amendment to the 1913 law, which would have allowed them to work students more than eight hours a day during their last year of training. Fortunately, the amendment never got out of committee.

Organized nursing, which always aimed for professional status, wanted to initiate its own legislative measures to control practice in their field. At the 1915 convention of the National League of Nursing Education some members raised questions about the events in California, speculating on whether or not they would be a threat to nursing's efforts to obtain the kind of legal controls that would enhance professional standards and growth. At the meeting much discussion focused on reports of various studies done around the country that had conclusively demonstrated the evil effects of long hours of labor for women in occupations other than nursing. In nursing particularly, one could demonstrate the connection between a shorter working day and alertness on the job. One speaker summarized the league's concerns:

> As far as I am aware only one state—California—includes hospitals and training schools, and controls the hours of duty for nurses as it does for women in factories. With this in view are we not in great danger of having the privilege of legislating for ourselves removed? Some other body seeing the ill effect of long hours of work for nurses may force us in other states by labor laws to conform to a standard which we should have ourselves recognized and established.
>
> One question for us to consider is—How can we place ourselves above and beyond the control of labor laws? As a nursing body we must recognize that shorter hours are demanded, and, could we not place in our state bills [nurse practice acts] a clause to that effect, thus putting our registered training schools above criticism and reproach? Then, as speedily as possible, should we not make our training schools comply with the educational requirements of colleges and universities, thus placing nursing on a professional basis. The term "pro-

fessional" can be applied in law only to a calling associated with a college or university, or to one where the degree of diploma is awarded through a college or university, or a chartered educational institution of that rank.[25]

These nurse educators did realize that their problem was basically an educational one. They acknowledged that under persistent conditions of extreme exploitation a law to regulate the working hours of students was warranted. It was at this meeting that Annie W. Goodrich had commented in part, "if our schools were really schools it would not be possible for them to be under any labor law," summing up the problem nicely.

These nurse educators also realized that they were nearly powerless to improve conditions in hospital schools. Indeed, improvements might well have been more speedily accomplished if the labor movement had further aided nursing in solving some of its problems, since the vast majority of evils inherent in the apprenticeship system were actually conflicts between labor and management. Nurses suffered from an almost total lack of influence over their own affairs. Hospital management was outside the bounds of any public authority and completely in control of policy making, and so conditions did not improve.

Hospital management was not sufficiently concerned about the quality of services provided by its labor force. Administrators gave scarcely any consideration to the selection of appropriately trained workers who were positively qualified to care for the sick. Prior to the 1930s there was no distinction made between the work performed by immature students and that performed by fully trained nurses. In addition, there was little intelligent attention given to an examination of staffing patterns—to have women working ten, twelve, and even more hours per day could scarcely have been a measure designed to insure quality or even efficiency.

In a paper published in 1919, Isabel Stewart presented some of the reasons why nurses themselves failed to accomplish more improvements of the conditions persisting in training schools. Stewart noted that nurses did not wish to be thought disloyal to hospitals and they did not want to "arouse public antagonism" toward their sponsors. Stewart maintained that the majority of nurses engaged in training-school work tended to identify with hospital management because they wanted to help maintain both the "efficiency" and "good name" of their employers.[26]

Apprenticeship, the system under which nurses trained, is the method of education most suitable for instilling a strong faith in superiors, a desire to cooperate, and a tendency to think less of oneself and one's own needs. For an apprentice nurse, the highly valued "integrity of character" meant fidelity to agreement, which encompassed traits of dependability and efficiency in carrying out assigned responsibility. These attitudes are desirable in certain circumstances, but being cooperative and agreeable, always denying oneself for the good of others and someone else's interests, can often lead to a lack of growth or to a state of stagnation in one's own sphere of influence and work. More often than not nurses, having faith in their superiors, were led to believe that working ten and twelve hours a day was their responsibility and necessary for the good of patients and hospitals. A few nurses, Stewart among them, were continuously critical of this practice and felt that these "scientific and humanitarian institutions" could scarcely afford to remain "so far behind many frankly commercial enterprises" in improving working conditions.[27]

Securing a shorter working day would not have changed the apprenticeship system, nor would it have ended any of the other means by which training schools exploited students and made a farce of the "education" they supposedly gave them. Apprentices were admitted in numbers large enough to meet the immediate demands for nursing service in the hospitals that maintained a school. Few qualifications were maintained and admissions standards were so lenient as to be nonexistent. Furthermore, there was no set time for admissions. Students were often accepted at any time in the year when a vacancy occurred in the ranks of those currently enrolled. As reported in 1923, it was a customary procedure to admit "groups of probationers three times, four times, five times, six times per year and not infrequently even oftener."[28]

This practice of increasing numbers of students to meet demands for immediate nursing service, regardless of the institution's educational or housing provisions, is illustrated by an outcome of the eight-hour law in California. Hospitals met the requirements of the law by simply increasing the numbers of students admitted to training. Thus, shorter hours in that state meant greater numbers of students, rather than an increase in the number of graduate nurses employed. Clearly, an eight-hour system in the schools did not alter the fact that pupil nurses carried the workload in the hospital. Hours were arranged and numbers increased so that students still provided the nursing care.

With hospital management in control of the school system and with no public body outside this group regulating apprenticeship practices, there was no numerical limitation placed on apprentices. Each hospital was free to meet its own needs with little regard to community or national need for nurses. Management responded only to the immediate forces of supply and demand in their own institution in determining how many or how few students they would admit to training departments. Few hospital officials gave any consideration to the effects this was having on graduate nurses and the society at large.

Although nursing as a branch of the health sciences continued to become more and more complex, some nurses, many physicians, and the majority of hospital managers held tenaciously to the position that apprenticeship was the best, if not the only, way to educate a nurse. In view of this argument, the educational provisions in schools of nursing were kept to a minimum. The decline of the social usefulness of apprenticeship training was of less concern to those with power in the health field than was their concern for their own commercially-based interest in apprentice nurses.

Lack of limitations on the number of women trained as nurses resulted in overcrowding and competition in the occupation, leading to the exploitation of both the public and individual nurses. Finally, lack of reform in the apprentice-ship system perpetuated a kind of educational preparation that was uniformly poor in quality and, therefore, unsuited to meeting social demands or changing health needs of the society.

The commercial value of the student to the hospital was at the root of many problems in nursing. Since nursing provided an essential service to society, the public did not for long escape the consequences of the exploitation of students, the resulting economic competition, and the circumstances surrounding a system of education for vital health workers that was not adequately designed to meet the needs of the times.

IV

Housekeepers
for the Sick

THE OFTEN INADEQUATE educational preparation received
through the unregulated apprenticeship system was rendered
worth even less because all "nurses," trained or not, competed
for the same jobs. There were few standards to evaluate nursing practice and no laws to control those engaged in it and
thus little value was placed on the education of women for
nursing. In effect, the training school system considered the
student as competent as the graduate. An untrained nurse
could, and often did, substitute for the trained nurse with
few questions raised about her qualifications. Graduate nurses
were forced to compete with students because hospitals used
students as their nursing staff.

The problem of young students competing with more
experienced nurses aroused the attention of the Society of
Superintendents of Training Schools even before the turn of
the century. A discussion at their national convention in 1896
revealed what these nurses thought of this situation. Graduate
nurses were especially critical of the use of students as a source
of revenue for hospitals. As one reported:

> Nearly all schools have directories for their alumnae. [But]
> accusations are often made by the latter that students are sent
> to the choice cases. Feelings of the deepest animosity and re-
> sentment are thus harbored against the school to its decided
> detriment.[1]

The alumnae directory was the method by which graduates commonly obtained employment. Hospitals maintained a list of the names of graduates and when families in the community called for the services of a nurse, graduates theoretically were notified. In practice, however, if a hospital sent its own students to care for private cases, they were sent to fill the jobs, thus graduates were denied an opportunity to provide their services for compensation. As a result, unemployment was a frequent problem.

Since the system worked as it did, with hospitals receiving compensation for student services and with hospital officials making the decision about whether to send an apprentice or call a graduate, the "finished product" was really in competition with hospital "raw material" for the slim economic rewards accruing from the practice of nursing. Hospitals not only controlled the system of education, they also controlled the employment system, curtailing job opportunities for graduates. As a nurse from Pennsylvania pointed out at the Society of Superintendents' meeting in 1896, "the competition of undergraduates with graduates" was not "fair". In her town, one or two students could keep four or five graduates unemployed for some time.[2]

The public was unaware of how the system really worked. For economic reasons, families were often willing to accept student services. Hospitals charged slightly less for this service than graduates charged. As one concerned nurse from Brooklyn, New York, put it, "it is an injustice when a nurse has graduated and gone out to practice, to constantly underbid her. Many people will take the pupil . . . because they thus pay five dollars less a week for the work."[3]

Surely the public would not have accepted sending young medical students out to practice medicine. Physicians themselves would not have tolerated such abuse of their professional standards. This practice did eventually decline, but more because the demands for student services within hospitals increased than because hospitals recognized the extent to which this practice took unfair advantage of both the public and nurses.

It would be difficult to determine the precise extent to which young students in training competed with graduates in practice, but that the competition was frequent is evident, though not highly publicized. This open competition between students and graduates for private cases in homes had less far-reaching effects on nursing and nursing education, however, than the almost universal practice, which continued until the 1950s, of using student nurses as the main hospital nursing staff.

The apprenticeship system was the basic reason for this. With the success of apprentice programs in the 1880s and 1890s, hospital attendants and domestic servants had been replaced by student nurses. The number of young women apprentices was regulated by each hospital's own need for nursing service. Every year greater and greater numbers of graduates were produced and sent out to make a living in private duty and public health nursing. The few graduates who remained in hospitals served mainly in supervisory positions.

Student nurse service cannot rightfully be equated with professional service. The fact that hospitals did equate them meant that hospitalized patients were often deprived of professional attention by fully trained and experienced nurses. Hospitals brought in a new crop of students every year and graduated the skilled nurses, and such turnover impeded any sort of organized effort by nurses to improve care. Trained nurses were deprived of an opportunity to systematically improve or enlarge the nature and scope of nursing practice within hospitals. The expansion and development of this role for nurses is recent. Many of the criticisms directed toward hospital care today derive from the lack of professional criteria applied in nursing practice.

Perhaps as after the fact rationalization, the status of the graduate in hospital nursing simply did not surpass that of the student, a problem that was the source of many conflicts and impediments to change within nursing. In 1913 Mary Alberta Baker, a superintendent of nurses at a hospital in Florida, presented her views on the comparative value of the graduate and the student at a national meeting of the American

Hospital Association. In setting forth the argument that pupil nurses were far superior to graduates in providing hospital care, Baker contended that a graduate "was not the equal of a third year pupil in the nursing technique and skill." According to Baker, the more experienced graduate did not display "any feelings of loyalty or devotion to the hospital, its traditions, methods or its doctors." In short, this superintendent of nurses supported the argument that the value of students to the hospital was superior to that of graduate nurses. In the discussion following Baker's remarks, other members of the American Hospital Association quite blatantly expressed prejudice against graduate nurses. They preferred students because they were "loyal to the institution" and "anxious to please" physicians.[4]

The question of compensation was part of the discussion: student nurses often did not have to be paid by the hospital. With the value of nursing service defined in economic terms, the argument that students gave superior care served as a convenient rationalization for continuing exploitation of both students and graduates. The quality of the care provided in hospitals could not improve under apprentice nursing service; students provided custodial care, carried out doctor's orders, and learned the skills to perform routine hospital procedures, but they were scarcely able to develop innovations that might have resulted in improved nursing care. Therefore, patients suffered under this system as much as did nurses. If the potential contributions of experienced nurses had been supported and encouraged in the early years of hospital development, health care delivery might have been organized in a more efficient, economical, and effective manner. Nursing care is still the major product dispensed by hospitals and when the quality of that care is poor the patient ultimately feels the effects.

The damage wrought on the quality of hospital nursing by the apprentice system affected other kinds of health care delivery as well. Since graduates were prepared as generalists able to work on any floor of the hospital, closing them out of job opportunities there forced them to seek employment elsewhere: in private homes, public health agencies, schools, industries, and social service clinics. Although hospital training was not designed to prepare nurses for work outside the hospital, graduates had to accept work where they could get it. Many were inadequately prepared to assume the responsibilities of industrial, school, or public health nursing. Here again, patients ultimately suffered. Few nurses were prepared well enough to capably transfer their skills to, or initiate improvements in, other kinds of health care.

Few health care policy-makers questioned whether hospitals, as narrowly oriented service agencies, could prepare workers for a broader social usefulness within the larger community. The perpetuation of apprenticeship for the economic advantage of hospitals failed to improve either educational offerings or the status of graduate nurses. Since their education was secondary to their labor, it seems that little value was placed on the quality of their training or on the kind of service they offered society.

Prior to the 1930s, there was a marked effort to devalue the skills and potential contributions nurses could make to the effectiveness of general hospital care. This devaluation carried over outside the hospital as well, but a hospital's treatment of its own graduates provides the most blatant example of discrimination against graduate nurses. Almost twenty years after Baker's charge that graduates were not suitable for hospital employment, hospital officials, including some nurses, still thought the services of students were superior to graduates. Many hospitals still did not employ even *one* fully trained nurse for the purpose of giving actual nursing care to patients.

The widespread acceptance of hospital apprenticeship did not derive from a demonstration of its educational or professional value in improving the quality of care provided patients, but solely from its justification in economic terms. Effie J. Taylor, representing the nursing profession on a panel discussion sponsored by the Council on Medical Education and Hospitals and the American Conference on Hospital Service in 1933, emphasized that the system of education was characterized by exploitation rather than by educational features. Taylor put it this way:

> The first objective of any professional school should be the education of the student for her vocation, and the service she may give should be incidental to her education for her profession. The fundamental objective of the nursing service of the hospital is the daily and immediate care of the patients, and all other functions should be secondary. But the primary function of the schools of nursing is in the hospital inevitably evaded. . . . In nursing schools even the apprenticeship system is exploited, since the major time of the student is spent in service with the minimum of supervision and instruction.[5]

Speaking on the panel with Taylor, C. Rufus Rorem, a Chicago physician and a member of the research staff of the Committee on the Costs of Medical Care, admitted that the superior status accorded students in hospitals was questionable. In his view:

> Hospital directors should not maintain too stoutly that a student is "as good" as a graduate, or even "nearly as good"; for, if the average technical and economic value of students approaches that of graduates one is forced to question the quality of education in the nursing school.[6]

Rorem clearly identified the inconsistencies in the thinking of hospital authorities and their nurse supporters in regard to the problems of nursing service created by discriminatory practices directed toward graduates. "To be sure," Rorem noted in his report, "a hospital director may frankly admit that his nursing school is a farce, but usually those who proclaim the economic and technical virtues of the undergraduate also uphold the paradoxical view that their own graduates are well educated." The real issue behind the insistence that students gave superior care was the comparative costs of undergraduate and graduate nurses. The major impediment to change was that it cost more to hire adequately trained nurses.

During the Depression, government agencies urged the employment of graduates in hospitals as a measure of relief for the vast number of nurses who could not find work in other kinds of nursing. Hospitals were encouraged to employ graduates at the same salaries paid to aides and practical nurses. Studies had shown that the latter groups, despite their having little or no training, were weathering the Depression much better than most fully trained nurses. The annual income of these nurse aides was higher than was the income of graduate nurses who did happen to be employed outside the hospital.[7]

The 1930s and the Depression did not signal the onset of an unemployment problem in nursing. It had been a problem since the 1890s. Since nurses were women, their unemployment was largely ignored by all but themselves. Beginning after the initial proliferation of training schools, nurses were forced to deal with problems of overcrowdedness and competition. The Depression served only to make the problem more obvious. At the same time government reaction promoted the misconception that unemployment of nurses was a temporary phenomenon, one common to many other professional and occupational groups during the Depression.

For some hospital leaders, the national economic crisis was just another excuse to maintain the status quo, to continue using the schools as a source of staff nursing. A president of the American Hospital Association, Paul H. Fesler, speaking at the convention of the two national nursing organizations in 1932, took the position that "business matters" in hospitals simply did not warrant the encouragement of "new projects" such as employing graduates or providing more educational advantages in the schools. Fesler warned nurses that physicians and hospital administrators would not support changes leading to the improvement of educational standards. He concluded that "each hospital has its own service problem" and arguments for change were destined to fail "when they meet financial barriers" in individual hospitals.[8]

Endorsing the status quo, another hospital administrator told a group of nurses in 1935 that "with economic conditions as they are for the public, for education, for hospitals there seems no chance immediately to change time-honored methods."[9] The Depression was used as a convenient rationalization for not improving nursing education.

Graduate nurses competed not only with students, but also with other partially trained and untrained women who were encouraged to fill the ranks of nursing. Almost as popular as the hospital school was the "short course" which provided a minimum of both formal instruction and practical experience. The short course was a short route into the nursing profession.

Short courses were offered by groups ranging from the Young Women's Christian Association to physicians who believed that nurses with less preparation than the hospital-trained graduate should be available to families of moderate or low incomes. The idea was to produce a worker whose fees would be less than those charged by nurses with three years of preparation. The often meagerly educated and apprentice-trained hospital graduate came to be thought of as a "luxury" beyond the reach of families with moderate or low incomes, and arguments were set forth in justification of the partially trained nurse. This category of worker gave rise to the concept of subsidiary workers in nursing. Eventually called attendants, aides, assistants, or practical nurses, their predecessors were the products of a short course operated under the auspices of anyone who cared to conduct one.

Some of the strongest advocates of the short-course nurse were physicians. In 1909, William O. Stillman, an Albany, New York, physician, proposed a rationale for two classes of nurses. Apparently arguing that the rich and the well-to-do deserved better care than the poor, he seemed to be reasoning that the kind and quality of nursing care made available to the public should be determined by their economic status. Speaking before the Medical Society of the City of New York, Stillman explained his point of view:

> [Few] physicians will be found who will deny the propositions that there is an urgent need for two classes of nurses. One must necessarily be the hospital graduate nurse. . . . But we

need another class of nurses who can meet the requirements and the purses of the masses of the people of moderate means. These persons constitute a very large majority of the population and it seems to me only fair and just that more moderate priced nurses, possessing a less perfect knowledge of nursing technique, and the conditions involved should be available for their use.[10]

Stillman had established his own course to produce "less thoroughly trained nurses." He told his audience that his "graduates" were encouraged to "restrict their charges to from twelve to fifteen dollars a week." "They are," he noted, "oftentimes offered much more." This physician urged fellow members of the medical profession to give greater consideration to the virtues of low-grade nursing care.

At its best, Stillman's plan was an attempt to meet a legitimate social need. However, his plan neither recognized nor considered what this worker was likely to charge in an open and competitive market where wages fluctuated and the public had no way of distinguishing between various types of nurses. In reality, "sub-nurses" served to make more intense the job competition in nursing. Moreover, the public, especially those with low or moderate incomes, did not get a bargain; families ended up paying the same rate for any and every kind of individual claiming to be a nurse.

One of the most ardent champions of the partially trained woman in nursing was Chicago's one-time commissioner of health, John Dill Robertson. Ten years after Stillman announced his proposal, Robertson established the Chicago School for Home and Public Health Nursing. His "school" offered an eight-week course and apparently produced thousands of "nurses." Arguing that only those of "very comfortable financial means" could afford hospital graduates, Robertson intended to solve the problem of insufficient nursing services for the citizens of Chicago by producing low-grade nurses. In explaining the success of his scheme, he reported that his school had graduated "790 in the first class and 1,363 in the second class" and he had hopes of admitting even larger numbers than this. Since women could move through the course in just two months, Robertson expected to have "train-ed 10,000 women" in one year's time.[11]

Conducted by the staff of the Chicago Department of Health, Robertson's course really prepared housekeepers for the sick, not nurses knowledgeable about disease or health. According to this commissioner of health, it was not necessary for his staff to attempt to teach "the meaning of symptoms." On the contrary, "throughout the course," he said, "we ham-mered on two main propositions—absolute adherence to the physician's orders and cleanliness." Despite such narrow prep-aration, Robertson insisted upon calling his graduates "nurses" and proclaimed that these workers were as compe-tent as hospital graduates in caring for patients with very serious diseases such as

> tuberculosis, diabetes and cancer cases; nervous invalids, el-
> derly persons, babies . . . any children's diseases . . . and in
> short, for the great bulk of nursing, these women are quite
> as capable as the registered nurse. Often they are more desir-
> able because they are willing to do housekeeping as well as
> nursing, and, in its final analysis, nursing is nothing more nor
> less than housekeeping for the sick.[12]

The association of nursing care of the sick with domes-tic service resulted in a devaluation of the nurse's need for specialized knowledge. Since nursing was thought to be meni-al woman's work, it required little expertise in its perform-ance. And yet, the public paid a fee for this service much higher than that paid for domestic servants—Robertson stressed the fact that his graduates worked for $15 to $25 a week, a price more like that charged by hospital graduates.

It was this type of thinking on the part of health care officials that resulted in grossly exploitative practices. Why didn't Robertson tell the public that his short course prepared housekeepers only and not nurses who knew about the symp-toms of disease and accompanying nursing measures necessary to help individuals recover from illness?

Obviously when people are sick enough to require nursing care, especially if they have "tuberculosis, diabetes, or cancer," they deserve more than a housekeeper. Families willing to pay for the services of a nurse thought they were getting a competent and qualified one, a nurse able to provide skilled care in time of illness. Moreover, at the time, if poor and middle-income families needed only servants and housekeepers, they could have obtained these services at a cost less than the $15 to $25 a week that they paid for Robertson's "nurses." Indeed, had these people been more informed about exploitative practices in the health field, many might have preferred to save their money. Other members of the family could just as competently have followed the physician's orders and observed the principles of cleanliness.

Even as renowned a physician as William James Mayo, one of the founders of the clinic that bears the family's name, was in favor of the proliferation of partially trained women in nursing. In comparing them with hospital graduates, Mayo argued in 1920 that the public needed "other types of nurses less highly trained but nevertheless important social service vehicles, the Fords, so to speak of the nursing world."[13] To implement his ideas, Mayo established a program in his hospital patterned after the Robertson plan and wrote articles endorsing the preparation of "sub-nurses." "Sub-nurses" was a term popularly used to describe the kind of worker advocated by physicians like Robertson, Stillman, and Mayo. The term itself has an interesting connotation, implying inferior status and preparation for a worker specifically intended to provide care for inferior members of society.

The practice of preparing sub-nurses was widespread from 1910 until 1930. Though hardly an egalitarian concept, the practice faced little opposition. Only a few physicians acknowledged the undemocratic reasoning behind the development of the idea of the sub-nurse. Richard Olding Beard of Minnesota, who advocated a high level of education for all practicing nurses, declared in 1913 that the "ends of social justice" could never be met by "the provision of graded nurses with training varying with the financial status of the employer."[14] Although proposed as a way to cut down the cost of delivering nursing care to poor and middle-income families, the preparation of "class A, B, and C" nurses resulted only in continuing exploitation of the public since all nurses, regardless of training, were paid about the same wages.

Despite its exploitation of the public and the already intense competition among hospital graduates, still another plan for training low-grade nurses became popular during the same time when short courses were prevalent. This was the correspondence course. Primarily a commercial activity, these courses produced uncountable numbers of nurses who claimed to be fully qualified, and sought private employment at standard rates of pay. Appealing advertisements led women to believe they could by way of "correspondence, secure a standing and training as a nurse, equal to that of the hospital graduate."[15] Thus, many women entered the job market as nurses without ever having attended a patient.

Most correspondence schools were actually "get-rich-quick" schemes. Their enterprising founders often offered physicians monetary rewards if they would recruit for such courses. Writing in the *Journal of the American Medical Association,* one writer urged his colleagues to beware of such untoward means of making money, reminding doctors that they might at some point be forced to engage the services of such so-called nurses. He said:

> It is the duty of physicians to discourage those who contemplate taking a correspondence course in nursing. In the end women so taught will be a disappointment to themselves, an irritation to physicians and a danger to the public.[16]

Although they were a danger to the public, correspondence courses remained a profitable business until the 1930s. Capitalizing on the ambitions of young women who wanted to enter a field in which they could immediately realize an income, these courses were advertised as "earn while you learn programs." Literature from the various "schools" indicated that applicants could earn $25 to $30 a week while taking a course of 24 or more easy lessons paid for on an installment plan. In the 1920s, the Chicago School of Nursing informed potential subscribers that they could earn not only these amounts but that many of the school's "graduates" earned as much as $35 a week. In addition, the literature indicated that recruits at the end of six months could earn "as much, or more money at nursing than graduates" of other nursing programs, including hospital schools.[17]

Sponsors of correspondence schools promised to furnish their "graduates" with certificate, cap, uniform, and a distinctive school pin. This paraphernalia paralleled that supplied to students in hospital programs, and in the public's mind gave the graduates of these diploma mills the same status accorded hospital school graduates.

The existence of correspondence courses and short programs for sub-nurses long constituted a severe problem. Nurse practice acts as measures of legal control in the various states that had enacted them were useless as a means of determining who could or could not practice nursing. No state until nearly 1950 had a mandatory licensure law in effect. Since the early 1900s permissive laws existed that granted registered nurses the privilege of using "R.N." after their name, but these laws did not prevent anyone else who cared to do so from practicing nursing for hire. This type of regulation really amounted to no regulation at all.

Since there were no effective licensing laws to certify those who practiced nursing for hire, commercial employment agencies opened to provide private duty nurses, particularly after hospitals stopped sending out their apprentices to fill these jobs. These agencies hired out most any woman purporting to be a "nurse," often charged exorbitant fees, and paid the nurse only a portion of what she earned. Had hospital registries for their own graduates been used to serve their proper purpose, there would have been little need for commercial agencies.

Amy M. Hilliard, superintendent of nurses at an upstate New York hospital, identified the prevalence of short courses as the major cause for the widespread existence of these agencies. Criticizing them at the 1922 meeting of the

American Hospital Association, she said that the commercial agencies freely engaged in

> the merciless exploitation of the public, the graduate nurse and attendant. If a purely commercial and unethical group get together and organize a registry, the temptation is for them to send untrained women out as graduate or trained nurses, in order that the percentage of money accruing to the registry will be greater. The women find it hard to resist the temptation to accept wages they are really not prepared to earn, particularly when this is coupled with the fact that the registries will call those more willing to go, if one refuses to be accessory to the fraud . . . much of the criticism for high nursing charges has come from this method of exploitation of the public.[18]

There is no record that the A.H.A. took any action to close down these agencies, though had hospitals made use of their own registries, they no doubt could have quite easily put the commercial operations out of business.

One of the more damaging results of the mass production of nurses by questionable educational programs was the constant assault on the occupational status of nursing. With standards of care so low and with the poorly trained constantly flooding the field, little could be done to improve the image of the nurse in the public's mind. A major consequence of the situation was to discourage many capable and qualified young women from entering the occupation. The demoralization of competent nurses served to drive many good prospects from the field.

The practice of preparing a worker less capable than the hospital graduate might have been more justifiable had it not been used as a means of lowering the status of legitimate nurses, allowing discriminatory conditions to constantly operate against them. Using arguments similar to those proclaimed by supporters of the apprentice system—that students were superior to graduates in hospital nursing—supporters of sub-nurses and correspondence courses proclaimed the virtues of the untrained nurse. Decade after decade, the most highly skilled nurses were forced into competition with the less well-trained.

In addition to facing oppressive economic circumstances, the nursing profession could not obtain the social status accorded other professional groups in American society. Would the public have been as willing to pay for the services of sub-doctors or sub-lawyers in competition with the more professional and better educated ones who were available? For that matter, in arguing for the full protection of the public and their own members, most professional groups through the use of legal and political action prevented the introduction of such workers to their ranks. In the predominantly female occupation of nursing, however, the choice of introducing or not introducing unqualified workers was not left to the profession itself.

With the greater influence on the legal and political system of its proponents, this argument against regulation held sway. It would seem that health care officials in and outside of hospitals were arguing that all women, regardless of educational preparation, should be allowed to practice nursing. As a result of this, the numbers of hospital trained nurses alone increased yearly far more rapidly than was warranted by increases in the population of the United States. The following statement from the final report of the Committee on the Grading of Nursing Schools, published in 1934, illustrates the extent to which the occupation was overcrowded:

> During the past 30 years the population of the United States has increased 62%, while the number of trained nurses has increased 237%. Approximately 100,000 new nurses have been added to the profession during the past 4 years.[19]

These figures, high though they were, applied only to hospital graduates, not to the correspondence and short-course nurses who were also in the job market.

Still another study, conducted under the direction of Harlan Hoyt Horner, then assistant commissioner for higher education in the New York State Department of Education, and also published in 1934, contains a cogent indictment of the system of education and the resulting conditions of over-crowdedness, competition, and demoralization among members of the occupation. Horner's report charged that the system responsible for the inexcusable conditions in the field was blatant commercialism. In his words, it was the attitude of hospital managers who maintained *"that profit may or ought to be made* [Horner's italics] out of a training school for nurses worthy of the name"[20] that was at the base of the problem. Such a system, the report charged, neither served the public nor provided nurses with a living wage. Unfortunately, this study did not investigate the other commercial activities in the health field, such as correspondence courses and the employment agencies, which seemed designed to profit from abuses of nurses and the public.

Horner's study of conditions in New York State did note that "weaknesses" in the apprenticeship method of education had resulted in "more than one vicious circle." In New York alone he found evidence indicating that the problem of the excessive number of unemployed nurses was not a product of the economic depression. For example, the number of nurses annually registered "increased from 12,524 in 1922 to 39,974 in 1933, an increase in 11 years of 219 per cent. . . . The number of nurses in active service increased from 17,850 in 1925 to 32,403 in 1933, or an increase in eight years of 82 per cent."[21]

Despite such increases, hospitals continued to admit large numbers of apprentices into their training schools. The demands for nursing service in hospitals kept business good and hospital officials continued to recruit students to provide nursing service. As Horner himself pointed out, though nurses were grossly underpaid, "the public complains of both the *cost* and the quality of the nursing service."

In conducting their study of the deplorable conditions affecting the quality of nursing care provided the public, Horner and his staff interviewed hundreds of patients and families to ascertain their views on the kind of care they received from nurses. Public attitudes about nurses constituted the greatest indictment of all against the method of training. The lay public was most critical of

> the inability of the average nurse to fit into the care of the sick in the home, and her ignorance of nutrition, contagious diseases, tuberculosis and mental diseases. Their comments dwelt more particularly and emphatically upon her want of culture, general education and social poise, and upon undesirable personality.[22]

Horner's staff also interviewed leading figures in the field of public health who employed nurses. They repeated the criticisms that families and patients had about nurses. In addition, these critics emphasized that the average nurse lacked a "preventive point of view," an "ability to teach the patient how to care for himself," or a "feeling of responsibility for teaching positive health." Thus, the average nurse was not equipped to provide the very essence of what constitutes nursing care. Sadly enough, when nurses were asked to evaluate themselves "their replies followed the same lines as those of the other groups approached."

In considering the low opinion of nurses held by the public during the 1930s, it is important to realize that apprenticeship systems of education in any society, at any time, have never been designed to impart either social graces or general education. "Culture" has always been the task of formal schooling in a liberal system of education. For this reason professional groups have sought to establish a place for themselves in colleges and universities; the nursing profession is no exception to this rule. But where other professional groups made rapid progress in acquiring a liberal education, nurses had to cope with hospital schools, eight-week courses training housekeepers for the sick, and correspondence courses. No other group claiming to be a profession since 1873 had to contend with such circumstances.

Health officials outside hospitals complained about the lack of culture and the unpleasant personalities of many nurses, too. But their colleagues inside the hospital system persistently maintained that these attributes of grace and learning were the very things that nurses did not need. Many insisted that the "average" nurse did not even need to learn the symptoms of disease, let alone learn how to teach patients about health and preventive measures. How could nurses teach what they were not allowed to know or assume graces they were not encouraged to acquire?

The poor quality of education received by the average student nurse and the lack of social and professional status of graduate nurses held them back from functioning effectively. As a group, they often did not know how to help themselves. Some nurse activitists did urge nurses to take constructive action to better their lot. One, Elizabeth C. Burgess, in speaking to her colleagues in the National League of Nursing Education in 1932, told nurses that they themselves "held back progress through their apathy, their lack of understanding, and because of their long domination by hospital interests."[23]

As Burgess noted, the nursing profession was itself "sick," suffering from an illness caused by the "medical and hospital care" it had received over the years of its life. The illness was acquired in infancy when nursing became the "stepchild" of the hospital family who saw "in this infant, money and service value." This illness, resulting from social pathology based on sexual discrimination and economic abuses in health care, had created a "vicious circle" of overcrowdedness, competition, and unemployment, with hospital schools continuing to swell nursing's ranks "with a stream of the incompetent!"[24]

The end of the 1930s and the Depression did not bring about significant reforms. Medical sexism, and its accompanying abuses of women, presented major impediments to changing health care delivery systems. By 1950, the economic status alone was deplorably low. Growing wiser, perhaps, about the social discrimination faced by a women's profession, many women refused to consider nursing as a career. Many already in the field left it for marriage or for better working conditions elsewhere. But the sick still had to be cared for and so women's refusal to assume servant roles resulted in cries of a "critical shortage of nurses."

National studies made in the 1940s showed that a widespread feeling of insecurity existed among all types of nurses. To escape this feeling, many nurses did turn their backs on nursing. Prompted by a "critical shortage" of nurses the Bureau of Labor Statistics, the Women's Bureau of the United States Department of Labor, and the National Nursing Council set out to investigate the conditions that gave rise to such shortages. Beginning in 1946, a series of surveys were conducted on the hours, earnings, and working conditions of nurses in private practice, public health, and hospital settings.[25]

Over 22,000 nurses responded to this series of questionnaires. Only one out of four nurses in institutional settings had retirement-pension plans, those limiting their practice to private cases had none. Many did not have any hospitalization or medical care benefits: "only two out of five nurses reported that they received hospitalization, medical care, or periodic physical examinations . . . only one out of six public health nurses received any such benefits."[26] Protection against sudden unemployment was almost nonexistent. Dissatisfaction over rates of pay, conditions of work, and promotions was prevalent.

Many nurses admitted that they worked only to supplement their husbands' incomes or, during the war, for patriotic reasons and because their husbands were in the military service. For women with small children, the burden of practicing nursing was even greater because they had to pay to have their children cared for. Many of these women worked only out of a sense of responsibility for the sick and suffering. The following comments by a mother with small children were typical:

> My children are small. Because of the shortage and the urgent appeal of the hospitals for nurses, I felt it my duty to hire a woman to care for my children so I could work evenings. . . . I had to be away from my home 6 hours, if there was no over-

time (for which we are not paid). All through the war I helped out . . . and cleared 30 cents for being away from home 6 hours. All this time our floors were laden to capacity— beds in the halls and an acute shortage of help. This situation existed until we had worked 56 nights; then our wages were increased to $3.00 so that we then cleared around 75 cents for an evening's work. What else but loyalty and community spirit would keep anyone working at a position of this sort?[27]

If nurses could clear no more than $.30 to $.75 for an evening's work, were not paid overtime or allowed rest periods in the morning or afternoon, it is not surprising that many decided after the war that they would be happier to stay home with their families. Nurses were women and, like good wives and mothers, were expected to be self-sacrificing for the weak, dependent, and the sick. Nursing provided few career incentives and those women who continued to work did so usually out of true commitment to the profession. Too, many had to work to support themselves or their families since nursing was for a long time one of the few jobs open to women.

High unemployment risk and job insecurity were problems that nurses continuously faced. These women were subjected to widespread public and private criticism for their lack of manners and knowledge. Deficiencies in professional preparation did not go unnoticed by those who employed their services, as clearly indicated by the Horner study. Through little fault of her own, the average nurse was simply not able to render very effective community service.

Apprenticeship education did not and could not provide a liberal education for nurses and it gave no attention to the responsibilities of citizenship or professional commitment. The education of nurses was a private matter controlled by the commercial interests of hospitals and this remained the case despite new concepts of health, the changing nature of social institutions, and the public demand for better educated nurses. The commercial basis of delivering health care was a major impediment to the realization of improved patient care. Student nurses were not prepared to meet community needs, but the needs of the hospitals as perceived by the hospital. Hospital officials failed to respond to new ideas about preventive nursing and medical care. They ignored the public's need for health education and their social responsibility to see that nurses were prepared to meet these needs.

Today nursing is still classified as a semi-profession. The numerous levels of practice, the structural complexity of nursing, has its origins in the early preparation of sub-nurses and other aides with varying levels of educational experience. In present health care delivery systems, aides, practical, technical, and professional nurses all work side by side, performing the same functions in many hospitals and other health care facilities.

Also, as a hangover from past practices, the most highly educated nurses are still discriminated against. Their status is seldom higher than that of the less well-prepared, they often have difficulty finding jobs in which they can function as professionals. Working conditions within hospitals are still poor. Seldom are distinctions made between either the functions or the monetary rewards granted the highly trained in comparison to those with less education. All this, of course, affects the quality of care provided the public.

Nursing's critics often know little of the causative factors or the historical background that has shaped the direction of its development. Contemporary sociologists recognize and are quite fond of analyzing the structural and functional complexity of nursing. Unfortunately, they are not quite so quick to recognize that nursing's social usefulness has not been developed to its fullest potential. One popular sociological finding, that nurses lack autonomy and work in an atmosphere of subordination to physicians, is hardly surprising to any nurse, but there is little she can do about it.

It seems that Americans are more easily excited by the notion of barefoot doctors in China than they are by what their own nurses could do with their shoes on. Despite the fact that many nurses now obtain bachelor's, master's, and doctoral degrees, the "bedpan image" still influences the public's attitude. Moreover, in many states, the law still sanctions the image of the nurse as one who merely aids the physician in his work or hospitals in their work.

Although more careful studies are being done on the work of the nurse, little information filters out to the general public. There is still little public recognition of nurses as professionals and nurses are forced to preserve the reputation of physicians and hospital administrators who entrust their "reputations" to them. Nurses have always assumed a great deal of responsibility for the delivery of health care. Though the public remains relatively ignorant of this, physicians and hospital officials do not. But only privately and informally will they give nurses the credit they deserve for their contributions. Their public support for nursing's improvement has never been, and is not now, strong. Instead, they have done much harm to the public image of nursing by associating it with domestic service or calling it mere women's work. To its own detriment, the public has not really examined the prejudicial myths underlying much that is said about nurses.

V

Sexism in the
Hospital Family

IN HIS ESSAY ON "The Subjection of Women," John Stuart Mill pointed out that systems of apprenticeship were ideal for keeping individuals subject to the will and wishes of others. Mill felt that the concept and oppressive use of apprenticeship were grossly incompatible with modern social ideas and institutions. Of the survival of apprenticeship, he wrote:

> that in all cases in which an apprenticeship is necessary, its necessity will suffice to enforce it. The old theory was that the least possible should be left to the choice of the individual agent; that all he had to do should, as far as practicable, be laid down for him by superior wisdom. Left to himself he was sure to go wrong.[1]

Freedom and competition were not permitted in older forms of apprenticeship arrangements. The preconception existed, in Mill's words, that "certain persons were not fit to do certain things" and thus, their activities were "authoritatively prescribed or dictated." These preconceptions apply quite accurately to apprenticeship education for nurses. It was ideal as a means of keeping a female group in subjection to male-dominated groups.

Nursing, perhaps more than any other profession, has been influenced by social conceptions regarding the nature of women. Modern nursing originated at a time when Victorian

75

ideas dictated that the role of women was to serve men's needs and convenience. Nursing's development continued to be greatly influenced by the attitudes that women were less independent, less capable of initiative, and less creative than men, and thus needed masculine guidance. In view of this definition of women, the education of nurses at the turn of the century was of special interest to men in the medical profession. The apprenticeship system was considered an ideal means of insuring that nurses so-trained would remain "ideal" women.

Hospital schools provided both a structural and a functional arrangement whereby the medical profession and male offiicials in the hospital could claim the right to exercise control over women. These two groups cultivated the idea that they had the "right" (and most often did have the power) to determine the direction of growth taken by a female profession. They repeatedly set forth arguments to support their view that nursing existed to assist physicians in their work and hospitals in their work. Writing in 1921 Isabel M. Stewart, one of the foremost nursing leaders in America, noted that this concept of nurses and nursing supported the "age-old tradition that men are naturally superior to women, that women exist mainly to serve the comforts and purposes of men, and that men know best what is good for women, whether in politics or education or domestic life."[2]

Education in American society has sought to bring about the freedom, equality, and independence of its citizens, but any group dependent on an apprenticeship method of education could not be expected to gain any of these at a very rapid rate. As a means of maintaining social and intellectual control over the nursing profession, members of the medical profession have been among the strongest advocates of this special, isolated type of education (or no education at all) for nurses. Physicians repeatedly expressed fears that nursing would gain its independence from medicine, and the medical profession. This fear has been traditionally revealed in the commonly expressed view that nurses did not need an education because the physician had one. "Womanly" qualities on the part of the nurse were valued more than knowledge.

Physicians, individually and collectively, spent a great deal of time attempting to convince both women in nursing and the public in general that nursing was subordinate to medicine and should remain so for the "public good." The "born nurse" theory was a popular argument supporting the contention that nurses were better off with little education. William Alexander Dorland, a physician and a member of the medical faculty of the University of Pennsylvania, expressed this widely held opinion in an address delivered before the 1908 graduating class of the Philadelphia School of Nursing. Urging nurses to accept the importance of their intellectual inferiority, Dorland warned:

> If a little knowledge is a dangerous thing in most avenues of employment, in nursing it is more than dangerous—it is fatal. Good nursing is not facilitated by too elaborate an education in professional matters; rather it is hampered or even rendered useless thereby. I believe that a superficial knowledge of physiology and anatomy, together with a thorough acquaintance with hygiene, will answer every purpose.[3]

Dorland went on to say "a nurse may be over-educated; she can never be over-trained." He minimized the need for education by commenting upon the "born nurse theory."

> If . . . a course of instruction in nursing is engrafted upon a fair general education, and this is backed up by a heap of good common sense, then may we expect to find a capable nurse—provided she has the nursing instinct. . . . A good nurse is born, not made.[4]

Dorland then elaborated on the notion that physicians should be regarded as superior in both knowledge and skill and that nurses should never aspire to such heights; for them to do so was not only "dangerous," it could be "fatal."

Dorland was not alone in expressing fears that nurses might become independent practitioners. In 1906 the following statement in the *Journal of the American Medical Association* urged physicians to place restrictions on what nurses were permitted to learn and do:

1. Every attempt at initiative on the part of nurses . . . should be reproved by the physician and by the hospital administration. 2. The programs of nursing schools and the manuals employed should be limited strictly to the indispensable matters of instruction for those in their position, without going extensively into purely medical matters which give them a false notion as to their duties and lead them to substitute themselves for the physician. 3. The professional instruction of . . . nurses should be entrusted exclusively to the physician, who only can judge what is necessary for them to know. . . . These maxims should certainly be borne in mind by the physician who has dealings with the nurse, as a matter of simple justice to her that she be not encouraged to take steps that are not in her province.[5]

Organized nursing's turn-of-the-century campaign to increase educational provisions in schools of nursing led some physicians to fear that nurses would become the equals of physicians in knowledge and skill and would thus usurp the authority of the doctor in the sickroom. In order to prevent this, the medical profession denigrated the importance of nursing education and warned nurses of the dangers inherent in their striving to go beyond a certain level of intellectual achievement.

It is understandable that physicians would object to the illegal practice of medicine by nurses. At the time nursing was a newly developing branch of the health field which was concerned about treatment, cure, health care, and the prevention of disease. Physicians diagnosed disease and prescribed treatment, but nurses, in constant contact with patients in homes, factories, clinics, and hospitals, provided the care and treatment for the acutely ill. Through case detection, nurses obtained help for those who needed it, and taught preventive measures to promote and maintain health. Nurses needed knowledge of the biological, physical, and social sciences as much as physicians did. In practice, they spent far more time with patients than did physicians and, in the absence of physicians, nurses made medical as well as nursing judgments in the management of patient care. Moreover, since physicians did not spend very much time with patients, they had to make some medical decisions based on data and observations recorded by nurses. If nurses were ignorant or poorly prepared, the patient ultimately suffered from errors in both medical and nursing judgment.

Prior to 1910 nursing was openly recognized as a branch of applied science that promised to be as important to the patient's health as did medical practice itself. However, despite the increasing responsibilities of professional nursing practice, the nurse's need for knowledge was greatly devalued and often denied her. The medical profession sought to eliminate competition with these women before their true value had been fully recognized by the public.

Writing in a state medical journal in 1905, a physician named Edward Ill emphasized that, with the exception of aseptic surgery, the trained nurse was the most notable "innovation in the practice of medicine" to be introduced in thirty years. According to him, the contribution of the nurse was so great that "many a practitioner would not care to practice medicine without her help." Notwithstanding this conclusion, Ill went on to praise "womanly" qualities in nurses—a "good" woman, and not education, made the best kind of nurse. As he put it, "the best all-around nurse is the good observer, the quick-witted, conscientious and resourceful woman. No amount of training will supplant these good traits."[6]

Physicians openly objected to the introduction of formal instruction designed to facilitate the provision of more intelligent nursing care. They favored nurse training that concentrated on the performance of routine tasks and were gravely concerned about preparation in scientific subject matter. With the introduction of formal courses, some physicians suspected that training schools were on the way to becoming "institutions for the higher education of women along medical lines."[7]

This charge was made by George P. Ludlam, a physician and the superintendent of the New York Hospital. Critical of the subject matter outlined in the curricula for some schools of nursing, Ludlam felt that the content being presented too closely resembled that found in institutions preparing men for the practice of medicine. Ludlam gave specific examples of the kind of thing he was concerned about. One course in dietetics was "sufficiently comprehensive to tax the ability of an expert analytical chemist." He thought this kind of teaching was "useless" since pupil nurses did not need to "talk learnedly on proteids, carbohydrates, starch, dextrin, minerals, and salts." Instead, he pointed out, the nurses needed to acquire an "appreciation of the importance of serving a piece of steak or a chop, hot and before the gravy has become congealed, or of accommodating the portion to the condition of the patient and the extent of his appetite."[8]

In an attempt to influence public opinion in favor of male superiority in the sickroom, two Philadelphia physicians, Henry Beates and William Alexander Dorland, organized a public meeting there in February 1909 to discuss the role of the nurse. Dorland set the theme by attacking the emerging leadership of the nursing profession. In an attempt to undermine public confidence in them, he criticized nursing leaders for their "autocratic" bearing and their efforts to impress upon nurses "the importance of their chosen calling."[9]

A formidable group of citizens had been corralled to hear this and other criticisms directed at the nursing profession. William P. Potter, a justice of the Supreme Court of Pennsylvania, presided at the meeting and declared that the subject under discussion was of vital "importance to the general welfare of the community." Beates, who was president of the Pennsylvania State Board of Medical Examiners, presented an address in which he emphasized that the nurse's knowledge should be limited to the barest essentials. He told his audience: "the instruction commonly prevalent in hospital training schools is not only absurdly too comprehensive, but dangerous. It is sufficient to almost entirely result in nurses assuming the right to usurp the functions of physicians."[10]

Both knowledge on the part of the nurse and legal recognition of her competence presented threats to the physician's authority. In Beates' opinion, nurses should cultivate a pleasant temper, cheerful countenance and encouraging demeanor, and be ready and willing to render those numerous and apparently small attentions which are of such great value in caring for the sick or injured, and which contribute so largely to an uninterrupted restoration to health. She should . . . never attempt to appear learned and of great importance. . . . In addition to these fundamental essentials, she should be able and willing to render intelligent obedience to the instructions of the attending physician, and carry out his orders to the letter.[11]

Advocating approval for these womanly attributes only, Beates informed his audience of public representatives that he did not think that the educational, economic, or legal status of nursing should be improved. Implying that it is not in the best interest of the public, he commented that the nurse as wage-earner, seeking a fee for service comparable to her training, was "not the 'angel of mercy' that she seemed to have been before training was established."[12]

The changing economic status of women was the real issue. Well-trained nurses were worth more than untrained ones. Fearing economic competition from women, physicians repeatedly complained about the increasing fees of practicing nurses. Many attempted to limit or at least influence the income of the nurse in the same manner as they did her level of education.[13]

Male supremacy had to be maintained by controlling women and keeping them in their place. Beates made a plea for an increased measure of control over nursing leadership. Arguing that hospital boards of trustees should "intelligently limit instruction," Beates stressed his belief that, "the education of the trained nurse for obvious reasons should be under the supervision of the medical profession; and hospital nurse superintendents and head nurses *especially*, the subjects of intelligent official control."[14]

The resolution that concluded the Philadelphia meeting stated that men in medicine should have "absolute authority in the sickroom, having control and direction of both the treatment and the nursing" of patients. Significantly, one clause in the resolution read, "nurses are not competent either by education or experience to be considered as consultants, or as having equality of privilege and duty in directing the affairs of the sick-room."[15]

Prior to 1910 the medical profession had reason to feel threatened by graduates of the more reputable schools of nursing. The course of study in the majority of medical schools was more narrow and more limited than that found in many nursing schools. Internships for medical education were not yet a common practice. Thus, physicians at the time were more than a little envious of the then "dominant" position of the nursing student in the hospital. Members of the medical profession were fearful that their "allies" in the nursing profession were well on their way to outdoing medicine in educational reform and professional accomplishment.

Male students had to compete with female students for learning experiences in the hospital and medical men resented this competition. In a speech delivered to the Medical Society of the County of New York in 1906, a physician explained the men's animosity toward women in the health field. He said:

> One obstacle between interne and patient is the modern training school system for nurses, which is absorbing for itself, through pedagogic ambition, a power and importance never originally contemplated by the medical profession.
>
> The overtrained nurse is expected to learn almost as much physiology, anatomy, and bacteriology as is required in the first year of a medical student's curriculum, and to spend at least one third more time in hospital service than does the interne. . . . It was recently discovered in one of our most widely known hospitals that an interne had been graduated without ever having given personally a hypodermic injection.[16]

That nurses were learning at the expense of medical students was considered a most "undesirable" situation. In an effort to eliminate competition and maintain the image of the physician as the "master" practitioner, some members of the medical profession adamantly opposed *all* educational reforms in nursing programs. Few could ignore the fact that trained nurses were improving patient care.

In a presidential address to the Indianapolis Medical Society in 1910, an Indiana physician expressed his conern that the "trained nurse proletariat" was being advised by their leaders to "assume the position of membership in a profession." His comments further reveal that he, with other physicians, had not originally realized that modern American nursing was bent on becoming a profession similar to medicine and law. Moreover, since medical men had not known of the nursing leaders' intentions, they had done little to "stop" early professional growth because nurses were plainly improving the care of the sick and "meeting the needs of physicians in the hospital and the home."[17]

As physicians realized that much of their success with patients depended upon the nurse, their desire to control nursing intensified. For nursing to continue along the lines of professionalization was perceived as a situation having "grave consequences" for the medical profession. Denying the full worth of nurses and the value of their contributions to the treatment, care, and recovery of patients perhaps relieved the insecurities of some physicians. Statements such as "The nurse is the handmaid of the physician, never his equal," "The best assistant is one who has never been educated as a nurse," "Heart qualities are better than the most elaborate training and skill," were repeated over and over.[18] A fear of competing with women seems to have motivated the opposition to the growth of a women's profession.

Medical men blamed themselves for having "permitted" nurses to become "educated" and "too independent." At a time when nursing, with all professional groups, was attempting to move away from apprenticeship, physicians expressed a strong desire to *stop* professional growth on the part of this group of women. Medical men were, no doubt, aware that an apprenticeship system with a minimum amount of formal instruction would serve to prevent or delay growth and progress toward professionalization.

The view that nursing was a subordinate part of medical practice, existing solely to meet the needs of physicians, became ingrained in the minds of the majority of men in the hospital and medical fields. The rank and file in nursing were persuaded to believe in their inferiority. Nursing students were repeatedly reminded of their subservient position and the system of apprenticeship by which they received their training provided no means for liberating their minds from this indoctrination. The very nature of training in hospitals prevented women from attempting to liberate themselves from the idea that they existed only to serve another group or institution. The political and social climate of the time was not yet ripe for women in nursing to create a different image in the public's mind.

Sexist and paternalistic attitudes toward nurses persisted. William Allen Pusey, the president of the American Medical Association who believed health care should not interfere with "survival of the fittest," commented upon the "proper" kind of woman who should enter nursing. In his presidential address to the A.M.A. given in 1924, he said:

> The proper work of the trained nurse does not contemplate that she is in a position of primary responsibility. Her duty is to care for patients' needs under the physician. . . . The work she has to do in ordinary service does not require a high school training nor three years of hospital training. It needs young women of character and intelligence, of a sense of responsibility and of elementary education. Given such a woman, and the time required to teach her in the hospital the technique of the nursing craft is a small part of three years.[19]

Pusey recommended even less training than had like-minded physicians a decade or so earlier. In essence, he wanted no more than domestic servants in nursing. He repeated the argument that nurses were born not made; any good woman would do, an argument still heard fifty years later.

Physicians were often puzzled by nursing's attempts to modify and improve upon the system of apprenticeship prevailing in hospital schools. W. S. Thayer, an earlier president of the A.M.A., indicated in 1920 that he could not understand why women might want to improve their educational status:

> Now it is a curious phenomenon that, as physicians are seeking more and more to abandon the classroom for the ward and the laboratory, those engaged in the training of nurses are tending to give more hours to the classroom and to complain that too much time is given to practical work in the wards, and this in connection with a training in which the practical side is of especial importance. One hesitates too hastily to criticize, but I wonder whether our friends interested in nursing education may not be headed in the wrong direction?[20]

It seems that Thayer did not understand, or at least refused to acknowledge, the existence of various problems in nursing schools. It was as though exploitation did not exist or at best was acceptable in the process of training young women. In his view, nursing should concern itself with the "practical" and the menial. Pleased with the quality of health care received by his patients, he was blinded to the fact that the scope of nursing practice went beyond the mere giving of physical care and cheery comfort.

This attitude presented insurmountable barriers to communication between medicine and nursing. Physicians argued that nursing existed only to serve them in a supportive role. In doing so, they devalued the contributions of women in the caring process and in the area of preventive health care. Notwithstanding the fact that nursing did perform a supportive function, as do almost all female groups in society, nursing leaders insisted that their profession had something to offer the public that went beyond the limited and often menial job of carrying out doctor's orders.

Sexist attitudes and paternalistic tactics on the part of physicians gave rise to a deep resentment on the part of nursing leaders. Nursing authorities did not think their profession was "merely a part of the medical profession" and they objected to the claim that physicians were responsible for improvements that had been accomplished by nurses.

Only a few prominent medical men spoke out against

the narrow-minded and repressive views of their colleagues. Winford H. Smith of The Johns Hopkins Hospital had as early as 1912 denounced fellow physicians and hospital officials for their opposition to advancements in nursing. Calling such activities blatantly "unfair," he reminded all that:

> The development of nursing has been the strongest of all factors contributing to present hospital efficiency, and this development has resulted almost entirely from the earnest efforts of members of the nursing profession, in spite of unwarranted opposition and in the face of adverse criticism.[21]

The dominance of medical education over nursing education in the hospital received official sanction in the 1920s when the Council on Medical Education of the American Medical Association officially became the Council on Medical Education and Hospitals. This change in title and focus came about because leading members thought it desirable for medicine to give closer attention to the ways in which hospitals could be used to the advantage of physicians.

At the 1925 convention of the A.M.A. the purpose of the Council on Medical Education and Hospitals was defined as the most appropriate means by which organized medicine could become more directly involved in the affairs of the hospitals. These institutions, it was thought, could provide "the solution of several of the modern problems in medical practice."[22] Almost inevitable in view of previous developments, the creation of the Council on Medical Education and Hospitals was an outgrowth of an historical process—early educational "connections" with hospitals had also enhanced opportunities in both medical education and practice. However, such connections did not serve, and have not served, as most favorable to the solution of the nation's health problems; nor did they enrich the educational climate for nurses who, with more opportunities and support, may well have been able to solve or at least prevent many of these problems.

With the formation of the new council, organized medicine arbitrarily decided to devote its attention to an intense consideration of how members could best use hospitals and nursing in the future. Since nursing schools were located in hospitals and nursing service was their chief product, the A.M.A. automatically assumed it had the right to make decisions about developments in nursing, as individual physicians had been doing for fifty years.

Thus, the 1920s and 1930s were witness to an unprecedented proliferation of committees on nursing appointed by the A.M.A. But, although they spent a lot of time trying, physicians themselves could not agree upon what was best for nursing. Completely ignoring the nurses' professional organizations, the A.M.A. through its own isolated deliberations set itself up as the nominal authority on nursing. The attitude that a women's profession and its services were a commodity to be used to the advantage of a male profession was given official approval and added impetus. The association's position on nursing as stated in 1927 was that:

> all surveys, studies and recommendations shall emanate from the American Medical Association and not from any newly constituted independent organization. The problem of nursing education and service is a vital one to the public and to every physician. It is a problem in which we should exert and evidence opinions and recommendations and accomplish their institution. It is a service we owe to the public, to hospitals, to training schools and to fellow members. The American Medical Association should, yea must, undertake its solution and formulate the resultant principles when they are announced. We become negligent and shirk our responsibilities and forfeit guiding direction if we delegate the task to others.[23]

Although medicine could "delegate" all kinds of "tasks" and the care of the critically ill to nurses in practice settings, organized medicine had no intention of taking any advice from nursing leaders. They seemed to assume that if women were left alone to improve the educational, economic, professional, and social status of the nursing profession, something drastic would happen to physicians' interests.

In a minority report presented in 1923, Richard Olding Beard, who first proposed the idea of university education for nurses, warned his colleagues that they were making a grave mistake by attempting to solve nursing's prob-lems alone. He raised objections to unwarranted medical in-trusion into the affairs of nursing and felt that the majority of physicians were not acting in the public interest or in a manner that would lead to the "ends of social justice."[24] Beard not only respected the rights of women as professionals, he also knew that these professionals were directing their efforts to improve training schools. Beard's concept of the nurse, which had led him to found the first university-affiliated school of nursing at Minnesota, was much more enlightened than that of his colleagues.

To be sure, much of what the nursing leaders were do-ing did not basically alter the system of paternalism they had to contend with. Their efforts did not result in lessening the economic exploitation of nurses or in changing commonly held attitudes toward women, but they kept trying. At the end of the 1930s, they turned their attention to problems in-herent in hospital control of training schools by increasing their attempts to obtain the cooperation of the American Hos-pital Association in bringing about reforms. Members of this association would not, of course, concede that the schools were used as a means of profiteering on unsuspecting young women. As Joseph D. Doane, president of the association and medical director of the Philadelphia General Hospital, said in answer to criticism of the hospitals in 1928: "It is a weighty obligation indeed to admit young women to training schools for educa-tion, but it is to me a far more serious thing to admit a sick man to a hospital unless he can be properly treated."[25]

Doane's concept of treating the sick must have been a rather limited and narrow one. Who administered treatment prescribed for the sick? Who cared for the patient 24 hours a day, observing his condition for sudden changes that could mean, depending on the action taken, recovery or death? The physician was not there to do it. Nurses did it, and was it not a more serious matter to lead the public to believe that care in hospitals was provided by a nursing staff of competent practitioners when in reality this was often far from the truth? Was it not a gross violation of the patient's rights to promise "safe" care and then not make it available? As one nurse educator, Effie J. Taylor, pointed out in a report on nursing education presented to a joint session of the Council on Medical Education and Hospitals and the American Conference on Hospital Service held in the 1930s, "one cannot but wonder that hospitals have been willing for so long a time to accept responsibility for a nursing service which . . . must inevitably be precarious."[26]

Despite the "precarious" conditions under which treatment was provided in hospitals, in Doane's view the "proper" treatment and care of a sick person was that administered by the partially trained nursing apprentice, and not a fully qualified graduate nurse. Could the apprentice administer safe, let alone "proper" treatment, when she, according to statistics presented by Taylor, received "direct supervision" for an average of only "eleven minutes per ten-hour day."[27] Quality in the treatment and care of patients has not been a priority of hospitals, despite the myths they have perpetuated. The myth that physicians supervise or have ever supervised nurses is just that—a myth. The lowly apprentice nurse was most often left alone to assume major unsupervised responsibilities for the care of sick men, women, and children.

Doane raised no questions about the quality of treatment or about possible ways of improving nursing care provided patients. Instead, believing that all women should ultimately become mothers, he argued that hospital schools were useful social agencies since "the profession of motherhood is certainly benefitted by the information, the knowledge, which nurses secure."[28] To commit themselves to a profession was not expected of young women in nursing. The educational activities of hospitals benefitted the public by preparing young women to be good wives and mothers, or so it was thought. Preparing women for motherhood and domestic life in the home was far more important than preparing them to care for the "sick man" in the hospital, let alone to make contributions in the fields of nursing and health care.

In 1935, seven years later, Doane made it clear that he had

> no apology to offer for the arrangement whereby schools for nurses . . . represent integral departments of the hospital organization. Nor am I asserting at the outset that this is the best plan. It is simply the scheme most frequently observed throughout the field and the one which in the light of our present economic difficulties seems likely to persist for not a short period of time. . . . Because hospitals, some by necessity and others through sheer blindness, have profiteered on this arrangement, their motives generally should not be impugned in any wholesale fashion.[29]

This was a familiar argument evoked to explain all: the system was to blame and individuals were not. One must, however, raise questions about some individuals and their efforts to discriminate against women and to maintain an oppressive social system that was harmful to both individuals and the larger health care system. Specifically, one must question the coercive manner in which domineering and more powerful male groups attempted to control, exploit, and interfere with the desired goals of a female group of lesser power and influence. As Doane reminded nurses at their 1935 convention:

> [for your] profession to endeavor to change conditions as they exist without the help of those others who should be interested, namely, hospital trustees, superintendents, the public, the patient, is . . . a hopeless task. The cause of the nurse may still be safe in the hands of that splendid army of trustees, many of whom need only to be shown the way.[30]

The suggestion that they collaborate with their oppressors could hardly have been welcomed by nurses who had been striving unsuccessfully since the 1890s to cooperate with that "splendid army of trustees." Such cooperative efforts aided the more powerful parties involved, the trustees. To them, the Depression was reason enough to continue the system of apprentice training for nurses, and no assurance was forthcoming that in a time of prosperity things would be different. Paternalistic attitudes and the system of structured inequality within hospitals were barriers to change not easily altered regardless of economic, social, and political changes in the larger society.

Some state medical societies joined with the A.M.A. and the A.H.A. in support of apprenticeship in nursing and denounced those student nurses who did not demonstrate sufficient "humility." The Michigan Medical Society's Committee on Nursing Service and Education announced this position in 1928:

> The Committee believes that nurses are overeducated. Whether it is the amount of learning or the manner in which it is acquired, it is more difficult to get the desired service from the higher trained nurses. The higher entrance requirements and the elaborate training given have helped to increase the cost of nursing. . . . The Committee recognized the following principles for endorsement by the state medical society: (1) nurses are helpers and agents of physicians, not co-workers or colleagues; (2) physicians should have a part in the direction of the training of nurses and in its limitations as should the hospitals which give the training; (3) the training of nurses should be simplified and the time of undergraduate training reduced to not more than two years; (4) the apprenticeship system must be maintained.[31]

Maintenance of an inadequate and isolated system of education for nurses provided a sense of security for both medicine and hospitals. They valued the attributes apprenticeship instilled in women because nurses so trained could be exploited without their making a public protest. Physicians could easily claim professional as well as male superiority over female workers prepared by apprenticeship. Furthermore, hospitals could more easily manage a nursing staff trained to conform.

The American public readily accepted the view that a well-educated doctor was "superior" to his apprentice-trained nurse. A poorly trained nurse could not be the physician's colleague, but she could be his servant or his "helper." Given the quality of education received by nurses, physicians did not have to compete with them or fear that they would challenge their competence. The apprentice system successfully kept women subordinate to a male-dominated profession.

For Lewis A. Sexton, an M. D. with "sexist" leanings, providing nurses with a higher education would be like educating "a people beyond their sphere of usefulness." Sexton wanted

> nurses who enter the profession for the love of the work and the good they may do: nurses who are willing to give of themselves to make the long, weary hours of illness less irksome; nurses the sight of whom is an inspiration and joy to all who may be unfortunate enough to need their services . . . the man or woman whose needs call for that gentle touch that soothes an aching brow cares little for a knowledge of the solubility of salicylic acid or the atomic weight of sulphur.[32]

Sexton's description of the nurse sounds more like a romantic ode to an "angel of mercy" than a 1931 report to a medical journal. Those aware of the responsibilities inherent in nursing work might well have worried about getting served the wrong kind of "acid" had they known that most hospitals were staffed by immature students with limited knowledge of drugs and solutions. Sexton, like those who practiced medicine thirty years before, placed emphasis on "womanly qualities," "humility," and self-sacrifice. The intellectual development of women made them less desirable as nurses.

The public, prior to mid-century, put forth little effort to support nursing education; though medical education was funded so that it could advance medical science, the women daily applying the principles of that science to social problems found little support for their efforts to gain knowledge of those principles. Paid for indirectly by the labor of students, the development of nursing education and practice have suffered accordingly.

Politically sophisticated and economically more powerful than nursing, the medical profession readily minimized and even eliminated competition from women in the health field. The nursing profession was clearly perceived as a group of women with the *potential* to engage in economic competition with men. The argument that women did not need an education because men had one stemmed from physicians' recognition that if nurses were well educated they might eventually demand a salary comparable to their preparation. Moreover, intellectual liberation could have led nurses to demand more equitable treatment from hospitals and their fellow citizens.

Despite nursing's long history, its social and professional status remained low. The economic status of this female profession failed even to reach levels achieved by more recently developed groups in the health field. The fact that nurses are women, however, is insufficient to explain why this women's profession has not made more progress in a field where it has assumed major responsibilities for a century. The lack of progress and accompanying low status may well have worked to reinforce the belief that women are naturally inferior and incapable of advancing to levels of competence achieved by predominantly male professions. Nursing's problems, rooted in the traditions of economic exploitation, inadequate education, and longstanding social descrimination, have plagued the profession for the greater part of its history.

VI

Action and Reaction

THE MOVEMENT OF NURSES to organize themselves was the result of feminine initiative, as was the establishment of the first hospital training programs. The introduction of formal training did not, however, change prevailing social concepts about women; Victorian ideas persisted. Twenty-seven years after the first hospital schools had been established, intellectual development was still thought to be harmful to a woman's normal growth and development, particularly to her ability to bear children. The notion that college women could not produce as many offspring as non-college women was widely accepted, even by physicians. The educated woman's tendency to "infertility" was the subject of an editorial appearing in the *Journal of the American Medical Association* in 1904. In its words:

> it is admitted that conditions of incomplete development of the genital organs in women are much more frequent than used to be the case. It would seem as though the intense mental application so freely encouraged by our modern educational system may very well serve to divert Nature's purpose of developing the sexual side of the being . . . it still behooves physicians to raise their voice in protest once more against the unnatural conditions that have developed and are unfortunately developing still more in our present day educational system.[1]

This attitude toward the intellectual development of women was characteristic of the time during which nurses began their organized efforts to improve their educational system. After training schools were accepted and widely established, nurses turned their attention toward the necessity of forming organizations that could guide developments in their young profession. Prior to the establishment of training schools, nursing work had been performed by untrained domestic servants. Developing nursing work as a profession engaged in by trained and knowledgeable women who could be socially productive and receive economic rewards for their efforts was of prime concern to early organizers.

By 1893, having improved the formerly deplorable conditions in hospitals, leading nurses wanted to improve the still deplorable conditions of disease and poor health in society at large. Prompted by their zeal to accomplish this social mission, nurses from several countries met together at the Chicago World's Fair to begin the tedious work of organizing women. In the spirit of international cooperation that affected the entire fair, prominent nurses discussed their plans. American and Canadian nurses agreed to form their association as a joint endeavor. A preliminary organization formed in Chicago determined that the first meeting of the American Society of Superintendents of Training Schools for Nurses of the United States and Canada (renamed the National League of Nursing Education in 1912) would be held in New York the following year. With the rapid proliferation of hospital schools, it is not surprising that the primary focus of this society was "furthering the best interest of the nursing profession by establishing and maintaining a universal standard of training."[2] An educational focus seemed imperative.

Although they identified the development of sound educational programs as their goal, the superintendents were equally concerned about the lack of legal status for nurses and the problems this presented in regulating those engaged in practice. As an outgrowth of the latter concern, society members at their first convention planned for the formation of a second national organization, one that could work toward obtaining a legal status for practitioners in nursing. This proposal became a reality two years later, in 1896, with the formation of the Nurses' Associated Alumnae of the United States and Canada (renamed the American Nurses' Association in 1911). The goal of the first was reform in education, the intent of the second was obtaining a legal status. The goals of both were to mutually foster the growth of nursing as a profession.

With the control of education in the hands of one organization and the control of practice in the hands of another, gaps in communication were inevitable. The lack of concerted action by both educators and practitioners created serious problems, as future decades were to prove. With this separation of functions, the foundation was laid for continuing lack of unity accompanied by conflicts and misunderstandings. The two separate organizations still exist today, and so do the conflicts and the misunderstandings.

For the sake of unity among nurses, and for the achievement of equal or complementary progress in both education and practice, a more politically sound plan would have been the founding of one organization, not two factions whose members would engage in disputes with one another from time to time, with little agreement on the direction of developments. This division of functions now seems particularly absurd since the founders of both were the same women who moreover did the early work of both organizations.

At their inception, the main difference between the two organizations was the envisioned composition of membership: superintendents of training schools in one, the body of practitioners in the other. Were their interests the same? Yes, and they were viewed as such at the time, but nurses were women, and women at the time had no political status. The burden of the task they undertook was, they felt, too great for one organization to assume. More realistic than men, perhaps, because they knew their intellectual development would not retard their "childbearing functions," still they were different from, and not the equals of, men in their organizational experience.

Though these early organizers may have been in error for establishing two separate groups within the short period of two years, still, for women, in their position, the work of establishing any group should not be minimized. At the very least, one can respect their identification of themselves as professionals, which they were in spirit and in action. Moreover, people are terribly prone to being victims of their circumstances and few are gifted with vision sufficient to foretell the future. Such was the case with early organizers in nursing. Their success in organizing at all prior to the turn of the century was a considerable accomplishment, though a step commonly taken by all groups bent on professionalization. Their difficulties in obtaining full professional status over the years, with recognition equal to other groups, should not lessen an appreciation of their intents and aspirations in the face of overwhelming obstacles.

Perceiving their work as extremely important for the public welfare and for nurses, they acknowledged the immensity of their undertaking. They approached their task fully aware of their inability to bring about change rapidly. M.E.P. Davis, in her presidential address at the third convention in 1896, expressed the attitude of members toward their powerlessness. They felt, she said,

> hesitancy and trepidation, realizing that in a way . . . [they are] quite powerless to bring about sudden or radical changes without the cooperation of the managers of the training [schools].[3]

Davis and her colleagues realized their helpless and dependent state as individuals with neither legal status nor political freedom. Organize they could, but controlling their own growth was not their right, nor would it be for decades to come. Their dependent status undermined their organizational efforts in many ways and was the basis of continuing defeats in attempts to bring about reforms. Their actions were characterized by appeals for support and approval to male-dominated groups in the health field. Though persistent in their efforts to obtain approval and support, it was not forthcoming, nor would it be in their lifetimes, or in the lifetimes of countless other nurses.

From the beginning, the nurses' associations were a minority group among nurses. The membership of the Society of Superintendents when formed was composed of less than a third of the total number of superintendents heading schools. Out of 221 schools in the United States and Canada by 1896, only seventy had superintendents who were active members.[4] Though the membership increased, this minority status continued to exist. In addition, other leaders in the health field, primarily physicians, established their own organizations and did not become members of a nursing organization, nor would they cooperate with one in improving standards.

Fearing failure because their membership constituted a minority, and in order to avoid antagonism and division among nurses themselves, members early agreed that assuming a "conciliatory" attitude was best. To "conciliate" and not "antagonize" were womanly qualities hardly sufficient for accomplishing the task they set for themselves. They were coping mechanisms only, and cope they did, for years. The men in the health field used this very attitude against them time and again to foster their own causes. Conciliation did not, moreover, serve to create unity among nurses themselves, but divisiveness. The conciliatory behavior of nurse educators in hospitals led to persisting antagonism and conflicts among educators and practitioners. Practitioners were especially puzzled when educators in California sided with hospital administrators and physicians who opposed the eight-hour protective laws that would have improved working conditions for student nurses. Thus, conciliatory efforts to avoid failure actually served to create a climate in which they would fail to accomplish their goals.

Identifying with reform movements of the day, such as the development of hospitals, for example, nurses saw themselves as "social reformers" and not as radical feminists, who were also active in the 1890s. This was not an unrealistic view of themselves, for nurses were "reformers" in the true sense of the word. This identification grew out of the fact that they had, through "public house cleaning" as they called it, reformed hospital care in America. When trained nurses, or more accurately women in training, entered hospitals, they

found dirt and disorder to be almost universal. Vermin and infection were common even in pretentious buildings. Immorality was frequent. Coarseness and vulgarity they often met, and went well armed with moral force and intrepidity. Extraordinary customs and conditions existed. In one beautiful and wealthy hospital, the morgue table was used for operations, though Lister had announced his theories. In another, all the small rooms built for special free cases were filled with the mistresses of the city board of aldermen. Management was poor, often, even when good intentions prevailed; nurses' working hours were from four in the morning until ten at night, with resultant slovenliness of detail, and night duty was almost always so defectively organized as to be practically non-existent. The trained women who plunged into this public house cleaning were so absorbed in it that to them, for a time, the outer world ceased to exist. It was quite as adventurous, quite as exacting, as war nursing.[5]

Having won the "war" against filth and immorality in American hospitals, these successful agents of reform revealed their aspiration to accomplish similar reforms in society at large. They envisioned their role as much broader than caring for the sick, and it was. Their role, even then, extended beyond the care of the sick to the health care of the well through prevention of illness. Graduate nurses functioned in communities, settlement houses, and other social agencies, not hospitals. Nurses were "social reformers" who had done a great deal for society since the humanitarian movements of the nineteenth century began. They were highly visible as useful women and this recognition made them realize how useful they were. Why shouldn't they want to do more?

Their self-concept as reformers was a theme in all of the writings of the early nurses. Mary Adelaide Nutting expressed the sentiments of the society at their meeting of 1897:

> The world has no interest dearer to it than the care of its sick, its suffering and its helpless; nor even though the fact may seem to be unrecognized has it any interest more important than the physical and moral improvement of its people. If our usefulness were limited to the former alone, one could hardly complain of scope, but add the duties of the [health] teacher and the reformer, and you place the profession of nursing at once where bounds can hardly be set to its possibilities.[6]

Perhaps bounds could not be set to the aspirations of these women, but bounds could be set, and were, to their professional growth. This group of women had "no interest dearer to them than the care" of the world's sick, but others in the health field did have interests dearer to them, such as hospital finances and commercial profit. Significantly, these organizers viewed themselves as the equals of, if not superior to, physicians in the role of caring for the sick. For, as Nutting said, a nurse like "the physician . . . touches the social fabric at every point. The reformations which she has brought about in hospitals . . . can be carried into every other condition of life where such work is needed."[7]

At the inception of organized nursing, nurses in many ways were the equals of physicians in their professional training and their contributions to the health care of society. However, they were not their equals in the political and economic spheres of human activity, or in influence on the public, and it was this lack of equality that would shape their development far more than their professional ideals. Economic, political, and derivative social factors impeded their progress, keeping their contributions and reforms to a minimum. Their economic value alone enabled more politically astute and commercially minded groups to grow and prosper at nurses' expense.

At the very outset, nurse leaders were not a "radical" group nor did they become one; they were busy caring for the sick. And the vast majority were not attuned to the ramifications of the problems women faced in a society where they had no political freedom, little legal status, and no right to become professional people. They also lacked a full appreciation of the extent to which more powerful male-dominated groups would attempt to stop their growth with little consideration of their ideals or potential usefulness. Their very necessity and usefulness operated against them.

In short, the basis of the problems confronting nurses was the relationship between men and women at the turn of the century. Underestimating this, perhaps because of their fears or because of their self-image as reformers, many leaders did not go far enough in examining the repressive atmosphere with which they had to contend in an effort to change the political, social, and economic status of women entering nursing.

From the first decade on, members of the two associations did not seem to fully realize what their problems were, nor did they publicly attempt to solve the problems they had in common with all women in society. Had nurses identified their problem correctly, and early enough, they might truly have become "social reformers" in the new century. Instead, their concentration on limited educational issues over which they had no control did little in the way of solving their problems or in elevating their own status or the general status of women. They did have educational problems, but a far more important problem was the social order in which women were dominated by men.

The 1890s, with its development of organized nursing, was a fateful period for the nursing profession. Leaders decided to preserve the apprenticeship system for training nurses, not as a conscious choice, but from force of circumstance. They made plans for developing a uniform curriculum to insure universally high standards in all schools. To lessen the hazards of narrowly specialized training given in small and special hospitals, which was a considerable threat to the educational system because of the growing number of these private, profit-making, limited-service institutions, they proposed cooperative efforts between hospitals to implement the concept of "affiliation."[8] Since nurses, like all women, were valued and employed for their versatility of skills, avoiding such specialization was essential if the main virtue in the apprenticeship system was to be preserved. Nurses hoped to reform a privately owned system of education in which they had no enforcement authority. They could not, for example, implement universally acceptable standards because each hospital school decided on its own standards. Still for decades nurses tried to achieve this goal.

In their earliest meetings, leaders discussed general practices that they found deplorable, such as the use of wages as a competitive measure to attract applicants regardless of qualifications, the selling of student services for the purpose of increasing hospital revenue, and the long hours of hard work harming the physical health of students. Finally, of major concern was the lack of theory provided and scanty amount of time allowed for classes, usually held in the evening when students were exhausted. Because of laissez-faire attitudes in the hospital field, these practices persisted for years. As a pressure group or a public force bringing about change, the nursing organizations were destined to have little immediate effect.

Because their primary focus was on educational problems rather than on reforming the social order itself, the talents of women in nursing were repeatedly stifled. Concerned about the physical, psychological, and moral nature of human nourishment in society, they should have been more concerned about their own in that same society. But the early leaders wanted, in womanly terminology, as one put it:

> To do all the good we can, in all the ways we are able, to as many people as we can reach; striving to our utmost to use our talents, not only in actually ministering to the sick, but in working for the general uplifting of human strength and of human character.[9]

Prior to the turn of the century, as nurses discussed the need for a "suitable code of ethics" as the "means of inculcating a proper professional spirit" among their ranks, other groups seemingly not so concerned about nurses' self-respect were also organizing. Five years after the establishment of nursing's first national organization, the hospital superintendents followed their example by forming the American Society of Superintendents of Hospitals in the United States and Canada, which was renamed the American Hospital Association in 1908.

Thus, in the same decade during which nurses conceptualized their potential contributions and talked of their plans for accomplishing professional goals, the organization for hospital managers met and talked of the business end of hospital development. From the beginning, the goals of the hospital organization were often in conflict with the goals and ideals of the nursing organizations. Managers insisted that hospitals were "business enterprises" and not solely humanitarian institutions. One of the founding physicians pointed out to charter members of the hospital association:

> the central controlling power, and the ultimate responsibility for the hospital, rests with the governing body, whether under the name of trustees, managers, governors, or what not.[10]

Organizers of the hospital association made no distinction between methods of management in private and in public institutions; their early deliberations eventually resulted in the establishment of a paternalistic authority structure in all types of hospitals, whether funded by public monies or private.

> While there may be a corporation or appointing power as in [public institutions] . . . it yet remains that the governors should always be the final and absolute authority, shaping the policy, regulating the affairs, and held responsible for the results.[11]

Hospital governing boards and trustees were composed

primarily of physicians and prominent businessmen from the community. It was these men who ultimately shaped policies and regulated the affairs of hospitals, including schools of nursing. It was these men who became policy-makers and boards of trustees for the American Hospital Association. And it is these men who should be "held responsible for" the resulting exploitation of women that grew out of the continuing operation of hospital schools.

With the formation of this association, the question of apprenticeship in nursing became, and remained, a business proposition. Nursing organizations had no power or authority to compare with that of the administrators and boards of trustees. The goals of professional training for nurses remained in conflict with the business end of hospital management and opposition to reforms grew out of this conflict.

In hindsight, it seems that nurses never totally recognized the strength of their opposition. A few realized that their singleminded efforts to improve educational programs were not enough to counteract the inhospitable circumstances confronting them. Critical of the society's "sporadic pieces of good work" and assistance in "various good enterprises," Lavinia L. Dock, a former secretary of the society who openly identified with the suffrage movement and actively supported the feminist cause, confronted her colleagues in 1903 with their lack of power and effectiveness. Charging that the influence of the group was weak, with little public force to bring about change on any widespread scale, Dock raised these questions:

> to what extent is the Society an influence? To what extent does it affect the public? How much does it actually guide nursing education? What weight has it with hospital managers and staffs? What amount of force does it bring to bear on its own members?[12]

The truth, Dock asserted, was that the society

> has not done what it might do; has not made itself a moral force; is not a public conscience; takes no position in large public questions; is not feared by those of low standards; al-

lows all manner of new conditions and developments in nursing affairs to arise, flourish, succeed, or fail . . .[13]

Much to Dock's dismay, most society members did not
openly identify with the suffrage movement or feminist cause.
In an effort to have the society become more outspoken on the
women's issue and other social concerns, Dock urged members to think in terms of their "latent" and "unsuspected
power" and the ways it could be used in an "intelligent and
energetic manner." Resentful of the professional injustices
and indignities suffered by nurses in their contacts with "over-
bearing" medical men and hospital managers, Dock reminded nurses that those who engaged in the continuing
abuse of women were neither friends nor benefactors of nursing or women. With some insight into coming events, Dock
told them:

> A quite determined movement on the part of certain of our
> masculine brothers to seize and guide the helm of the new
> teaching is . . . most undeniably in progress. Several of these
> same brothers have lately openly asserted themselves in print-
> ed articles as the founders and leaders of that nursing educa-
> tion, which, so far as it has gone, we all know to have been
> worked out by the brains, bodies and souls of the women to
> whom this paper is addressed, and who have often had to win
> their points in clinched opposition to the will of these same
> brothers, and solely by dint of their own personal prestige as
> women.[14]

Dock was, of course, too much of a radical feminist for
the majority of the leaders in organized nursing. Ignoring her
warnings, the society went about the tedious details of trying
to formulate plans for improvements that did not involve public or political activism on social issues as such. The "latent
powers" of which Dock spoke were to remain latent. Acutely
aware of their dependency on the good-will of managers,
medical directors, and boards of trustees in private ownership
and in control of the schools, leaders had no intentions of
antagonizing these groups at the very outset of their work.
Trained nurses had prestige, recognition, and visibility; there-

fore, the necessity for radical public action seemed unwarranted to the majority. Although they would in less than a decade, nurses had not yet thought of moving away from privately owned schools to collegiate education for their profession.

   Before nursing organized itself sufficiently to cope with its increasing problems, the American Hospital Association, along with physicians, had organized their opposition to any reforms in nursing education and practice. And, in the first decade of the century, many nurses began to actively cooperate with the hospital association, a factor serving to further divide the energies of nurses.
   In partial explanation of this cooperation, the superintendents of the schools also served as nursing service administrators in hospitals. Since graduates did not practice in hospitals at the time, the concerns of educators were primarily for student welfare and not for the welfare of graduates, for improving conditions in apprentice programs, and not for the status and employment of graduates, or for the development of practice outside of hospitals. As a result, misunderstandings between educators and practitioners were inevitable.
   By being a part of local management in hospitals and by going along with management's official organization, the American Hospital Association, the actions of early leaders gave rise to the gap between nursing education and practice that has not yet been bridged by unified and meaningful cooperative efforts on the part of nurses. Initial efforts of the training school superintendents to cooperate with the hospital association actually began in 1908 and 1909 with the formation of the A.H.A.'s Committee on Training Schools. Members of the nurses' Society of Superintendents were asked to participate in the work of this committee, which they did. As committeewomen they gave their input to that association's organized efforts to intensify its control over the schools and the standards that should or should not be met.

In this joint effort, dealing with a subject of much concern to them, their service as committeewomen very shortly led to their absorption into that association. During the second decade of this century, the superintendents of the schools actually joined forces with their oppressors by becoming associate members of the hospital association. At this level of membership, the women had no voting power and no influence on the policies of the organization, though nurses were able to present their problems at meetings of the association.[15]

This involvement of nursing leaders may also be explained in part by the nature of administrative lines in hospitals and the subservient position of the nursing superintendents in this hierarchy. Since the schools were run quite undemocratically, the superintendents, just like students, had to abide by the rules of the hospital administrators and boards of trustees. Responsible both for the care of patients as well as the welfare of students, they had to subordinate the needs of the students to those of the hospital. The superintendents, in their joint appointments as nursing service directors and as heads of schools, could not experiment, innovate, or make changes without the approval of their superiors. Given this situation, they sought approval for their plans by use of their own "personal prestige as women," as Dock put it. They also used this approach in attempting to bring about reforms which led to their becoming nonvoting members in their opponent's association, a position that did not advance their cause at all.

As one member explained at the national convention of the society in 1910, three years before any of them joined the hospital group:

> in the hospital training school we have conditions unlike any other school. The presence of a large number of dependent people [the sick and women] would seem to preclude the possibility of any experimentation. . . . The training school is not an independent organization. It is most intimately bound up in the hospital, its association with which is an essential factor of its existence. The hospital having taken the responsibil-

ity of these sick people, rightfully demands that proper care be given them and certain punishment follows on neglect and carelessness.[16]

The superintendents themselves were subject to "punishment" if they should "neglect" patient care in favor of improving conditions in the schools. The care of the sick was a burden they took seriously. They, like students, had to engage in

recognizing rightful authority and obeying orders unquestioningly. The same discipline that inculcates these virtues in the raw recruit will undoubtedly foster them in a woman if used by the hospital where she is training.[17]

Having received training in hospital schools themselves, the heads of the schools acted with the same spirit of respect for rules and obedience to authorities they had learned as students. Restraint, discipline, and, of course, indirect and not direct action to bring about improvements was demanded of them by the conditions mandated by hospital management. The paternalistic system, whereby the hospital was the "guardian" of the schools and the women in them, whether students or superintendents, enforced compliant behavior both within the schools and in the organized efforts of nurses. Maintenance of this restrictive environment was supposedly necessary for the good of patients, or so it was argued.

Hospital authorities provided housing for students and permitted the superintendents to exercise limited authority in the operation of the schools, but both had to make concessions and give back much in return for their privileged existence within these institutions. In exchange for support, protection, guardianship, and their very survival, it is not surprising that interpersonal relations both on an individual and an organizational level were characterized by compliance with those in superior positions.

By 1910 paternalistic reactions on the part of physicians were quite as evident as those on the part of hospital managers. Much of this reaction had to do with the formation of the nursing organizations. Physicians did not want nurses to organize and they objected to the nurses' claim that they could be a profession. In 1910, a physician by the name of Thomas E. Satterthwaite declared that the main problems in nursing were the fault of the small number of, as he expressed it,

> women, possessed, I am sorry to say, of inordinate ambition, and having improper conceptions of the relative position they hold to physicians on the one hand and to patients on the other. They have injected into nurses' associations ideas that are erroneous and full of danger to the nursing community . . . while we as physicians have failed to recognize the grave consequences of the movement.[18]

In their efforts to organize their profession, nurses were criticized for being disloyal to patients, when in reality their organized efforts were intended to improve patient care through the ultimate improvement of nursing education and practice. Satterthwaite associated the organization of nursing with poor quality in patient care. For this he blamed independently minded nurses, saying "the nurse is the handmaid of the physician, never his equal . . . loyalty to the physician and faithfulness to the patient do not form a twofold proposition but a single one." This physician, like many others, equated a nurse's disloyalty to a physician with disloyalty to patients, an argument that is still alive yet a century old. Satterthwaite revealed his real concerns when he emphasized that the actions of organized nursing had "gone far toward erecting nursing into a profession like that of medicine, but controlled by women nurses."[19]

Dock's perception of the intents of their "masculine brothers" in the medical field was quite accurate. Not only was the hospital association to persistently oppose reform in the training schools, members of the American Medical Association began their own movement to impede the growth of nursing as a profession and the efforts of organized nursing to solve the problems in their system of education. With these two associations working to counteract their efforts from 1900 on, the difficulties faced by nurses intensified.

At their 1911 convention, and at almost every convention held thereafter, members of the Society of Training School Superintendents identified the system of paternalistic controls as the major impediment to nursing's progress. One member stated the problem well when arriving at the conclusion that nursing by degrees had passed from ecclesiastical control

> over into the control of hospitals and the medical profession ... under that control ... [nursing] has been strictly subordinated to hospital and medical needs.[20]

Concerned with the new significance of nursing to changing ideas about "the conservation of health and the prevention of disease," society members discussed the increasing need for better educated nurses who could fill positions in non-hospital agencies such as social service clinics, public schools, and industries. With their awareness of the changing role of nursing, and its expansion into various institutions other than the hospitals, leading nurses concluded that the hospital could not meet their educational needs any longer. What nurses were seeking was "the opportunity to know enough of the truth to serve all humanity, not in one hospital or groups of hospitals, but to make their fullest contribution to the world."[21] Still wanting to bring about reforms in health care outside hospitals, nurses were increasingly dissatisfied with their educational system.

At their 1911 convention, the nursing superintendents also discussed their need for public support of an education within colleges and universities instead of just within a private system that entailed no public financing. Between 1900 and 1920, various attempts were made to bring about the development of formal relations between hospital programs and educational institutions for the purpose of supplementing apprentice training. Since many hospitals did not provide even elementary science courses, many superintendents of nursing schools thought of turning to the high school, a state-supported public school created to meet community needs at the expense of property owners. They firmly believed that some public funds, or a different sort of private endowment, should help hospitals educate nurses for community use. They found, however, that in too many cases high school courses in chemistry, physics, sociology, and economics were terribly elementary and not at all what nurses needed. One committee exploring the possibility of using high school courses found that practical subjects in domestic science were of little educational value and were said to be designed for "incorrigibles or incompetents."

Furthermore, the nursing superintendents found that some high school principals thought girls of eighteen and nineteen were not "old enough to study about social conditions in a community, and should not be confronted with such harrowing problems as child labor, industrial disease, delinquency and crime, prostitution and drunkenness and the agencies by which society deals with these conditions."[22] The principals were ignoring reality because, as the investigating committee of superintendents put it, "the young nurse will meet these things at the very threshold of the hospital . . . and she ought to be ready to look at them sanely and in relation to the whole."[23]

And so the nurses' association turned to technical institutions, to colleges and universities, again falling far short of success. Preparatory courses at the Drexel Institute in Philadelphia and at Pratt Institute in New York, established in 1903, failed soon after they opened, as did courses at the Kansas State Agricultural College in Topeka and at the University of North Dakota. Isabel M. Stewart, the author of many books on the history of nursing as well as an authority on nursing education, wrote in 1918 about attempts to establish preparatory courses in connection with colleges:

> The success of such courses had not been very promising. . . .
> The time proved, as a rule, too short to get any great advantage from the college connection, the course gave the student no definite academic standing. Hospitals offered very little, if any, inducements to students taking such work, and since

the additional training was usually optional, and taken at the student's own expense, it is not perhaps surprising that so few took advantage of the opportunities offered.[24]

With colleges offering no academic standing for courses and hospitals not encouraging them to attend, student nurses had little reason to assume any financial burden for their unrecognized efforts. The predominant control of hospitals in this field of education perpetuated apprenticeship training of a rather primitive nature—learning by being moved from one hospital floor to another. The introduction of formal instruction within the probationary period was one attempt to capitalize on the initial phase of training when new recruits were of least economic value to hospitals.

Initially introduced in only a few hospitals, this formal instruction during probation was the first significant educational feature developed in the system of apprenticeship. It was not, however, either widely or rapidly accepted by hospitals. Although formal courses were first introduced in 1893, by 1923 they were still being experimented with by leading schools. In the 1920s, the initial phase of training was still a time for hospital authorities to examine students as to their physical fitness and ability to endure the hardships of the term of service. Formal courses did not become a common feature in nearly all schools until the 1930s.

Most hospital authorities were even opposed to the idea of affiliation between hospitals for the purpose of supplementing apprentice training—the method proposed by the nurses' association as a means of preserving the generalist preparation they needed in their practice. Hospitals opposed affiliation because they feared that broadening student experience would lead to feelings of disloyalty to the home institution. In 1908, a physician and member of the American Hospital Association expressed a view held by many for decades:

> Affiliation with other hospitals is a matter of serious import. It may engender dissatisfaction and discontent because the pupils are meeting with different conditions, different and often conflicting rules and regulations, and the peculiarities

of different supervising nurses. The feeling of loyalty to the interest of any one institution is hard to create. We send our nurses out for obstetrical experience . . . but there are grave difficulties in the plan.[25]

For a period of thirty years, officials of both small and large hospitals fought against the use of affiliation, an innovation that did not involve any basic alteration of the apprenticeship system. Some administrators feared that it would undermine loyalty to the home hospital; others objected to the added expenses and the sacrifice of student service while they were in another institution. Some simply objected to the disadvantage of having to make the necessary adjustments required in arranging additional experiences for students outside their own hospitals.

In spite of management's opposition, leaders in nursing steadily insisted that affiliations should be established as a standard requirement in programs not providing content or experience in areas essential to the general practice of nursing. To them, affiliation seemed the only reasonable means by which apprenticeship could be effective in preparing a relatively competent nurse. In 1916, Ella Phillips Crandall, a member of the Committee on Education of the National League of Nursing Education, presented a strong argument in support of affiliation to members of the American Hospital Association. She argued that affiliation was the only way to meet the economic needs of the hospital for nursing service and, at the same time, to provide a generalist training for nurses. In the hopes of gaining the approval of hospital officials, Crandall told them:

> such affiliation can be established without injustice to the hospitals or the communities which they serve. While much prejudice against such affiliation still exists, it is unquestionably the only solution of the economic need of student service and a standardized educational requirement.[26]

With versatility of skills required by nurses because of the nature of their work, they had a right to this provision in the apprentice programs. And yet it was not forthcoming in most schools until the 1950s. Spokesmen representing hospital management continued to argue that standards in education should be subject to the laws of supply and demand in order for hospitals to meet local needs. As justification for poor standards, or no standards at all, this argument is illustrated by the outcome of a meeting of the executive committee of the Hospital Conference of the City of New York, held in January 1912. Reacting against efforts of organized nurses in that state to require one year of high school prior to admission to a hospital school, the committee argued that this requirement had created a "dearth of pupils" and placed a "hardship on hospitals which are conducting properly equipped and ethically administered training schools."[27] Insisting that standards be kept "elastic," hospital managers asked for a freer hand in defining the proper way to operate their schools.

No doubt management's argument that a low entrance requirement was for the "public good" served to mold public opinion to the attitude that the actions of nursing leaders were harmful to that same "public good." However, organized nursing was neither unaware nor ignorant of the needs of the sick or of hospitals and attempted to initiate only those reforms that would not negate these needs. Thus, Crandall, in her efforts to persuade hospitals to accept the requirement of affiliation, specifically emphasized in 1916 that this minimum standard, if observed by hospitals, could "be made to provide approximately equal advantages to all students of nursing without disturbing the balance of supply and demand in hospital capacity in any community."[28] Presenting proposed reforms in a tone of appeasement was typical of the manner in which organized nursing approached members of the hospital association, otherwise they probably would not have been permitted to speak on the various issues.

Dependent upon hospitals and physicians for support, the work of organized nursing had a built-in tendency to failure. In 1912, at the national nurses convention, Mary Jean Hurdley, superintendent of the University of Virginia Hospital School at Charlottesville, spoke in favor of public support for nursing education. Realizing that apprenticeship would last as long as the public expected nursing education to support itself, she pointed out that

> nowhere, and at no time, have higher educational institutions, or institutions which prepare for life work, been self-support-ing. To prepare a lawyer, a doctor, or a nurse to efficiently render service to society, society must pay a part of the costs.[29]

In Hurdley's view using the faculty and facilities of existing educational and medical institutions would lower the operating costs of nursing programs and prevent wasteful duplication of effort. For

> *that* which is needed for medical training is just *that* which is needed for work in the Training School. One of the great evils of public education is the *needless* and extravagant duplica-tion of teaching plants, and it is just as culpable to waste the energy and money of philanthropy as it is to waste the money of a state . . . the money of both belongs to society and should be conserved.[30]

But Hurdley and her colleagues were dealing with deeply ingrained prejudice against their sex. Educating wom-en for a profession was not a priority in the health field, nor was it a public priority. Although, by the second decade of the century, apprenticeship had proved to be a socially inef-fective way to educate a nurse, authorities and the general public still insisted that it was the only proper way to do so.

During the time period when the National League of Nursing Education formulated plans to improve educational standards, members of the Nurses' Associated Alumnae (later the American Nurses' Association) sought to obtain legal rec-ognition for practitioners. Opposition to this organized effort was just as strong as the opposition to educational standards: the legal recognition of nurses (strict state registration and licensing laws) was associated in the minds of many with the issue of women's suffrage, and incurred heated resistance.

Despite the association with suffrage, the two issues were rather separate ones. Women's suffrage dealt with the

issue of political independence for women, whereas the registration of nurses was an effort to obtain legal recognition of
nurses as persons trained and qualified to engage in the care
of the sick. A male nurse, for example, could not obtain legal
recognition anymore than could a female one prior to the
movement to enact nurse practice laws. The whole issue of
registration for nurses had little to do with the fight for wom-
en's right to the vote.

Registration was a professional and an educational issue. Nurses themselves did not identify their problem as a
women's problem. Instead, their efforts were limited to the
single issue of having trained nurses rather than untrained
nurses recognized as the only people allowed to give nursing
care for a fee. Though the nurses' movement did take place
during the same period when women were struggling to get
the vote, the two movements were not related or coordinated.

Nurses merely wanted the social sanctions and protection accorded other professional groups. Since nursing was,
along with medicine and dentistry, one of the first three organized professions in the health field, nurses wanted to be
recognized just like dentists and physicians. This was reasonable enough, but here again they overlooked the basic problem that they were women, and therefore, without the right
to realize their ambitions. Since they were second-class citizens, they were destined to become, by enactment of the early
and ineffectual nurse practice acts, second-class professionals
as well.

The full connection between the right to vote, a status
independent from men, and professional status comparable to
men was not seriously considered by early leaders in their
push to obtain control of their educational programs and practice. Education and narrow professional aims got in the way.
Nurses obtained legal recognition as they intended, but this
recognition did not obtain for them the freedom to function
independent of men as professionals. Instead, the laws only
made more evident the nurses' subservience to the physician.
So even though nurses fought much opposition and obtained
a legal status very early, the laws merely institutionalized in-

equality between nurses and physicians. The state nurse practice acts gave public sanction to this continuing inequality.

Thus it has always been, as John Stuart Mill, in an
essay on the equality between the sexes, so cogently noted:

> from the very earliest twilight of human society, every wom-
> an (owing to the value attached to her by men) . . . was found
> in a state of bondage to some man. Laws and systems of polity
> always begin by recognizing the relations they find already ex-
> isting between individuals. They convert what was a mere
> physical fact into a legal right, give it the sanction of society,
> and principally aim at the substitution of public and organ-
> ized means of asserting and protecting these rights, instead
> of the irregular and lawless conflict of physical strength. Those
> who had already been compelled to obedience became in this
> manner legally bound to it. Slavery, from being a mere affair
> of force between master and the slave, became regularized
> and a matter of compact among the masters, who, binding
> themselves to one another for common protection, guaran-
> teed by their collective strength the private possessions of
> each, including the slaves.[31]

Already bound to hospitals through apprenticeship
with its guarantee of support, guardianship, and protection,
legal recognition for nurses bound them to the authority of
physicians. The recognition they obtained was that of practicing nursing under the supervision of physicians, and no
more. This legal subjection to authority of physicians has persisted into the 1970s. Only a few states to date have enacted
new nurse practice acts that recognize nurses as independent
practitioners; the vast majority have not. Thus, the legal system has repressed nurses quite as effectively as the educational system. In reality, many nurses have always functioned
independently as professionals, but most do not because it is
illegal for them to do so.

By incorporating the inequality of physicians and
nurses into law, the nurse practice acts gave legal sanction to
medical sexism: men were to supervise women whether they
were in the presence of these women or not. This supervision
was then, and is still, literally an impossibility in many cases

because physicians are not present in most of the settings where nurses are engaged in practice. Maintaining the independence of men and the myth of women's dependency through legal recognition of a status difference is rather plainly prejudice against women.

Moreover, the early legislation did not, as it should have for the protection of the public, deal with the real social necessity of distinguishing between the trained and the un-trained who practiced nursing. The absence of this provision in the laws was due simply to economic considerations. The commercial abuse of women could be more readily engaged in since no laws existed to prevent or curtail it. The legal status of nurses provides only one example of the double standards existing in the health field for male and female practitioners. Medicine and dentistry did not for long have to cope with the totally untrained entering their field as competitors who worked to destroy decent standards of practice.

Until mid-century and after, with a rare exception, organized nursing did not achieve legal provisions that effectively regulated practice. Literally anyone could engage in nursing if she wanted to do so. New York was the first state to enact a law that effectively controlled all women who engaged in nursing practice for compensation. Called a "mandatory" as opposed to a "permissive" law, this legislation, though passed in 1938, did not go into effect until 1947.

Opposition to mandatory nurse practice acts in the various states came from hospitals, physicians, commercial employment agencies, and those conducting short and correspondence courses for nurses. Since hospitals owned the schools, nurses pleaded with members of the American Hospital Association for support on this issue. Despite their pleas, a majority of the A.H.A. remained overwhelmingly against placing any legal restrictions on those who practiced nursing for hire. The hospital association opposed all legislation that might serve even indirectly to influence those admitted to training schools.

Instead of supporting the nurses, the public hospitals

joined forces with commercial hospitals and correspondence schools in openly opposing constructive changes in laws regulating practice. They refused to support such legislation on the grounds that it was class legislation and therefore undemocratic. Since such legislation already existed for other professional groups, the claim that this was class legislation was hardly applicable to the case. Since it aimed to eliminate abuses and exploitation of the public, the claim that it was undemocratic makes little sense.

After the First World War, when the apprenticeship system was again on firm ground, physicians increasingly expressed their disapproval of and their animosity toward nurses. They argued that the nurse should remain "a true physician's assistant" and should continue as a "household helper" in the homes of the sick. "For her own good," they wanted her to "be a little more human" rather than seek higher standards and legal protection. All she needed to know was how "to write, to read, to reason."[32] In 1923, the House of Delegates of the American Medical Association concluded that the nursing problem had become a "vexed question" and that the nurse should "remain a trained lieutenant of the physician." Their increasing hostility toward nurses in the 1920s was a reaction to the registration efforts and higher recommended standards set forth by the National League of Nursing Education.

At the national convention of the American Hospital Association held in 1929, Richard P. Borden presented the views of boards of hospital trustees toward nursing education and who should control standards. Emphasizing that hospital trustees were in the "business" of maintaining health, Borden's argument was:

> Who is to determine what the standard shall be? Is it not true that the parties primarily interested and therefore qualified to judge are physicians and hospitals, under whose direction nurses must perform their duties? The physician wants a nurse qualified to do what he requires of her; the hospital wants nurses to do nursing work in the hospital. The busi-

ness men, transformed for the time being into a hospital trustee, would spend no money in educating nurses in subjects which do not yield a proper return on the investment.[33]

Borden expressed well the decades-old attitude toward education for nurses. It was this attitude with which organized nursing had to deal. In doing so, leaders in nursing spent little time organizing nurses to take public action against the repressive forces of vested interest groups. They knew of the deplorable conditions confronting every practitioner in nursing, whether trained or not, but they took little public action to correct the situation. Instead, they continued to work privately on their problems and during the 1930s even increased their efforts to "cooperate" with the American Hospital Association.

Identifying the "need for a closer working relationship with the American Hospital Association," members of the National League of Nursing Education "offered the cooperation of the League" in efforts to solve the nursing problem, a public problem at the very least. Forgetting that their past failures had stemmed from this co-option of their efforts, the League in 1939 established a new "Committee to work with the Nursing Committee of the American Hospital Association," with a physician as its chairman. At the League convention in 1936, a report of the committee indicated that a "most pleasant and happy relationship" with other members had been established. Moreover, nursing members believed

> that the relationship which has been established through this joint activity has done much to bring about a better understanding of each other's problems and has emphasized the importance of still closer cooperation between our two associations.[34]

This reaction to the work of the joint committee indicates the extent to which these women believed in the goodwill and improved intentions of the hospital association. Without examining the history of their problems adequately, they repeated past errors unknowingly. Their search for support, for "happy" and "pleasant" relationships with men, although deemed necessary for the care of the sick, wasted their valuable energies, which would better have been devoted to communicating with the public and practitioners in the American Nurses' Association to mobilize their support for changes in the educational system. This was especially indicated since both hospital and medical groups had little intention of cooperating with nurses.

Members of the National League of Nursing Education finally realized in 1940 that they were not going to obtain support from medical and hospital groups, and in that year, they established the League's own accrediting committee to evaluate and determine the standards that should be maintained in programs of recognized caliber. This was a significant development because it was the first time in the history of nursing that nurses decided to make their own policies and control their own standards in schools they approved, with or without the support of other groups. One can only speculate on what might have happened if nurses had taken this step in the first decade of the century by identifying their problem as a women's problem.

When nurses did attempt to exercise control over educational matters, members of the American Hospital Association offered adamant opposition. They, as usual, wanted their organization to have equal representation and voting powers on any and every committee dealing with the question of nursing standards. The hospital association refused to approve the League's accrediting program. The nurses refused to grant them official representation on their accrediting committee. In response to their demands, League members simply replied that their bylaws "would permit only members of the League to be eligible" to serve in an official capacity on a standing committee of that organization.

Taking the step toward controlling standards did not, however, end the controversy. The 1940s continued to be a decade of conflict and turmoil between the three largest groups in the health field, all over nursing. Medicine intensified its efforts to look into the nursing situation and the House of Delegates of the American Medical Association declared in 1945 that:

> The problem is so definitely one of multiple jurisdictional interest and responsibility in which the medical profession as well as hospital management have a major part and obligation to the public to use the weight of their experience and authority in assisting to bring about the most perfect program possible in the nursing field.[35]

It was this type of authority and this type of influence that had led to abuses in nursing and exploitation of the public. Such authority had not provided solutions; it created problems instead of solving them. As public spokesmen for nursing and on issues in health care, physicians and hospital authorities have maintained their controls in this vital area of public concern. Not informed of the real issues and problems surrounding health care, the public was a victim as much as were nurses.

Greatly influenced by Victorian ideas about women, nursing leaders seemed intent to remain "ladies." That they accepted many of the Victorian notions of subservience is reflected in their writings and shown by their actions. Though acutely aware of their problems, they assumed a conservative approach to solving them. Conciliatory attitudes and behavior, along with their heavy responsibilities and duties in caring for the sick, prevented any accurate analysis of their real social and political problems as women dealing with a system of paternalism.

VII

Nursing and Health Care

HOSPITALS THROUGHOUT OUR HISTORY have been businesses operated with little, if any, economic planning. They have been conducted as local, private institutions rather than public ones and the development of medical-teaching hospitals only served to intensify this proprietary spirit. The development of complex teaching hospitals did, in fact, increase the opportunity for physicians to profit from the conduct of these institutions, free of government interference. As a result, the social mission to provide quality health care for all who need it has been considered secondary to economic and educational functions.

If the American people have been persuaded to believe that hospitals have always existed to serve the public in the best way possible and that this has been accomplished, they have surely been persuaded to believe in a myth. The public for too long has trusted in the leadership of powerful and outspoken professionals in the health field and has relied heavily upon their assessment of society's health needs and the means by which these are to be met.

Problems surrounding the American health care system derived from a process of historical development that has its roots in changes and events that occurred in the early part of the century. Today's concerns have been concerns of the past as well: there are no controls on costs or quality in hospitals; administrators and physicians remain more concerned about their own interests than those of their patients; hospitals and doctors are accused of profiteering in the health business at the expense of the public good. Moreover, there is no national health policy nor any efforts toward national planning for health preservation; provisions for quality and social economy have been either ignored or defeated, largely by private interest groups, of which the American Medical Association is a prime example. Health has remained a private matter and has yet to become a public responsibility.

The root of the problem, of which nurses in particular have long been aware, is that in the past and at present the needs of the hospital as opposed to the needs of those whom it serves have preoccupied the minds of powerful leaders in the health field. Despite the sometimes antisocial tactics used by physicians to maintain their control, sociologists and the public have idealized them, helping them maintain their public image as the perfect professionals.

Although organized medicine has both created and perpetuated social problems of major significance, the public is still encouraged to accept medical paternalism and to look up to doctors as final authorities on matters of health and illness. Historically physicians have demonstrated a narrow interest in disease itself and have devoted less attention to the social and psychological conditions giving rise to disease.

Nurses traditionally and currently assume responsibility for most of the care given to most of the people in almost every health care facility in the country. Physicians are often just not on the scene to assume this responsibility: an hour's surgical procedure, however essential, or a five-minute visit daily does not compare to the unique function of the nursing profession in its efforts to maintain continuity of care all day long, day after day. The continuing professional vigilance of nursing is indispensable to insure the recovery of patients who have received medical diagnoses and are taking prescribed treatment.

Nursing is health care. If current and future crises in the health field are to be resolved effectively, society must face this fact. More than a hundred years ago Florence Nightingale emphasized that the scientific laws of health and of nursing were one and the same. Today, another eminent nurse has pointed out that "the goal of nursing as a field of professional endeavor is to help people attain, retain, and regain health. The phenomena with which nurses are concerned are man's health-seeking and coping behaviors as he strives to attain health."[1]

If health care is of national importance, the nation must become concerned about the status of women providing nursing care in the nation's hospitals and elsewhere. All too often professional nursing attention is not available in many hospitals. Without good nursing service, quality care cannot be obtained regardless of the medical labeling of disorders and the prescribed treatments dictated by busy physicians. Health care cannot be adequately understood without an examination of the role of women in providing care. Nursing as a women's profession has been oppressed for a century and many of its problems merely reflect society's attitudes about women in general.

The role of nursing in the health field is the epitome of women's role in American society. Not accorded full professional status or an opportunity to obtain it, the nurse is viewed as a working female who is not expected to make a life-long commitment to her career. Like health care itself, the development of the potential of women's contributions to the betterment of society have not been a priority consideration in the United States. Nurses' efforts to obtain an education and professional standing have been impeded. With educational programs isolated in locally and privately controlled hospitals, nursing did not get public interest or support for its development. The financing of nursing education through the use of public funds is a recent development and the amounts of these funds are still meager in comparison to those provided many other groups.

Since nurses are primarily women, traditional perceptions of their role have in no small way influenced the kind and quality of nursing care given, and the extent to which this care and the means of its distribution could be improved. Received in hospital schools rather than in institutions of higher education, their preparation for nursing careers has not only been inconsistent in quality, but has stifled initiative by rewarding subservience.

Caught in circumstances they could not easily alter, nursing leaders have done their profession and the public harm by acquiescing to male-dominated groups in the health field. Second-class professionals, they have functioned as second-class citizens as well, not communicating openly with the public. Though representing a silent majority in the health field, these leaders, themselves invisible and faceless to the public, have not viewed political activism as either a virtue or a necessity. Since health care has always been highly influenced by local politics where the powerful tend to win, women's lack of sophistication and less than aggressive leadership has remained ineffective in bringing about favorable changes.

Despite the background of severe obstacles, nursing as a profession has made considerable progress since mid-century. Nursing has now established standards and national accreditation for all schools of nursing, controlled by the profession. College and university preparation for professional nurses is now widely accepted, but not yet a universal reality and debate over the kind and quality of education needed by nurses continues. Not until 1965 did the American Nurses' Association formulate its first position paper on nursing education. The association took the position that "minimum preparation for beginning professional nursing practice" should be a baccalaureate degree education.[2]

That organized nursing waited until 1965 to come out with such a policy statement reveals the extent to which the apprenticeship system has been viewed as essential to keep hospitals functioning efficiently, and to produce the bulk of nurses. Even now, physicians, hospital authorities, and some nurses still continue to oppose the closing of hospital schools, maintaining that these institutions provide the best means of meeting manpower needs in hospitals.

A significant innovation in nursing education has been the development of associate degree programs in community colleges. Such technical education for nurses probably accounts more for the closing of hospital schools than any other factor. Had these associate degree programs, supported by public monies, not been successful, the movement toward closing hospital schools would probably not have become a reality at all. The establishment of these community college programs provided a means by which nursing manpower needs could be met while decreasing the number of hospital programs.

Despite this innovation in nursing education and the increasing number of university programs, influential medical authorities still maintained that hospital schools must be continued for financial reasons alone. For example, in 1966, one year after the American Nurses' Association published its position paper, physicians asserted that these university educated nurses would become faculty members, visiting nurses, and administrators, not nurses who would staff hospitals and provide direct care to patients. Prominent physicians conceded that universities might in time assume responsibility for supporting nursing students in the same way they support medical students; however, in their view, this change in policy and tradition should occur slowly, if at all.[3] As of old, arguments against nursing's movement into educational institutions emphasize that the quality of patient care will suffer if nurses spend too much time learning the "theory of nursing." Medical men still argue that there are dangers inherent in the tendency of nursing educators to allow time for the acquisition of knowledge; an advancement, they say, which is not in the best interest of the nursing profession.

Perhaps nursing educators have not yet achieved an ideal solution to the problem of how to combine practical work experience and formal education, but this is a common problem of concern to many educators and professional groups, medicine included. Although skills are important in any practice, it is the knowledge base and the research contributions that enable a profession to meet the changing social demands made on it. Both the public and educators need to consider the dangers inherent in forms of education that meet only the service needs of hospitals as defined by management, the narrow focus that medicine would like to see nursing maintain.

Although hospitals were identified as educational institutions and were said to have been "community" oriented, this was defined as the community within the walls of the hospital, a limited definition that did not lead to a concerted effort to examine the goals of the institution in relation to its responsibility to the larger community or the nation as a whole. Hospitals still maintain a narrow focus and for this reason nursing can scarcely revert to closer educational ties with these institutions. Too much remains to be accomplished in the health field for nurses to move backward instead of forward. The apprenticeship system of training produced nurses who could not question the status quo. Thus, they fostered defects in existing practices.

The education received by nurses in privately controlled service institutions was oppressive and paternalistic, greatly influenced by the institution's own traditions, rituals, and parochial concerns. The power structure in these hospitals was authoritarian, a system that best served an elite few, often functioning to the detriment of staff and patients. Questions of authority and accountability are those needing the most crucial consideration in nursing and health care at the present, yet few nurses think to question the power structures in which they work. They have more often than not supported vested interest groups instead of looking out for their own needs or those of hospital patients or the public in general.

Both nurses and the public need to examine problems of authority in health care delivery systems. Nursing has been traditionally defined as a "supportive" profession, more so because nurses are women than for any other reason. Prior to 1910, nurses were more certain of their independent functions in the health field than they are today. Before the introduction of skilled nursing in modern hospitals, patients often went to these institutions to die. In lowering mortality rates, nurses were not performing the discarded functions of physicians: they were practicing independently their own profession and, in doing so, saved lives. They wanted to be instrumental in bringing about reforms that would benefit society as a whole by an emphasis on preventive health care. But the emphasis of national policies has been disease and not health, which has resulted in a lack of support for nursing.

Physicians, through their position of authority in hospitals, have perpetuated this emphasis on disease. With nursing more or less bound to medical authority, it has moved slowly toward a concentration on health. Today physicians still assume that nurses will remain in their "logical place at the physician's side" functioning "under the supervision of physicians" for the purpose of "extend[ing] the hands of the physician," statements of the American Medical Association's Committee on Nursing approved by the association in 1970.[4]

Unfortunately, well-qualified nursing service directors and head nurses of hospital units who attempt to bring about improvements in patient care are too often dismissed from their jobs with little cause or reason given. One head nurse in an Illinois hospital was recently fired from her job because she did not wear her white cap while on duty one day. The cap, an outdated symbol of purity, dignity, and the innocence of an angel of mercy, could hardly be called essential to the performance of her duties in caring for patients and handling administrative responsibilities. Such symbols and myths signifying the subservience of women no longer serve any useful function but serve as impediments to growth and change.

Other myths more consequential than the white cap bind nurses. One is the myth of medical supervision. Nurses do not practice in the presence of physicians and are not constantly supervised by them. Nursing care goes on without either the consultation or the presence of the physician. Absentee supervision by physicians is a reality in practice that ought to be recognized by law. Current controversy over the role of women in society should help nurses gain public support to alter outdated legal controls over the "right" of nursing to function as an independent group of professionals, separate from medicine. It is time that society recognized both medicine and nursing for what they are, two separate professions, different from each other, but both offering essential services.

Research done in a 1968 study on the quality of hospital care found that patients expect very little from the nurse and view her decision-making competence as minor in comparison to that of the physician. Patients preferred the attention of the physician even on matters within the domain of nursing.[5] Both patients and nurses suffer from this devaluation of the nurse. These findings can be duplicated in practice settings more than five years later, and provide evidence of the harmful effects of medical paternalism. Nurses, whether male or female and regardless of the level of their educational preparation, are limited in what they can do for patients. These observations of nurse behavior are clearly an outgrowth of the traditional views physicians have expressed about nurses. The desirability of the nurse maintaining an "inferior" position is a "good" only in the mind of the physician, it is not a good for the nurse or the patient. The public in wholesale fashion, has reinforced the paternalistic attitudes of physicians without realizing their ultimate effect on the care given in hospitals.

Historically American physicians have enjoyed one of the highest and most respected positions in society, but they misused their privileges by failing to institute cost controls or support comprehensive health programs. They have tended, instead, to favor the interests of hospitals, other physicians, and commercially-minded groups, rather than the interests of the public or the nurses on whom they depend.

Physicians seldom perceive nurses as anything other than the women with whom they work and nurses relate to physicians not only as a nurse to a physician, but as a female to a male. Patients are not encouraged to trust the judgment of nurses and nurses have little incentive to make judgments that are either disregarded or limited in their effect. For any real improvements to occur, the public must make a distinc-

tion between what the physician has to offer and what the
nurse has to offer. Quality in health care will not improve
greatly until distinctions are accepted and endorsed by both
physicians and the public, whose attitude toward nurses
will be changed thereby.

Medicine and nursing have not constituted a complementary "pair" of professional groups having common goals
and interests. Though both developed in close proximity, this
has not resulted in either effective communication or cooperative activity for the good of patients. Medicine has passed
tasks down to nursing as medical practice has become more
highly developed and technical, but physicians have not been
willing to communicate with nurses to learn their views about
who does what in health care and why.

Traditionally most nurses have accepted their unequal
status without critical appraisal or public action to change it,
an attitude fostered by apprenticeship. Nurses have also hesi-
tated to become the patient's advocate since they are limited
in the extent to which they can influence the patient's welfare. Thus, patients have been left without anyone to look out
for their interests in a system that is confusing to the average
lay person and dependent upon the good will of health care
officials.

Nurses should direct public pressure toward the form-
ulation of national health policies that will insure the full
utilization of their abilities and talents. This will require that
some attention be given to the image of the nurse, which is
damaged by media presentations depicting nurses as women
in white who follow doctors around. The public is misled by
this portrayal of the nurse's role and by news media that seldom provide information on new developments in nursing.
Reports on innovations in health care may mention nurses,
but only peripherally. It is essential that nurses attract more
favorable attention to their role in health care, if the public
is to utilize them appropriately.

The image of nursing is also damaged by another major problem requiring the attention of the public and nurses.

The problem of control that organized medicine exerts over nursing does not encourage the public to explore better ways of utilizing the services of nurses. Medical men appoint themselves public spokesmen for nursing. As public spokesmen, medical men have perpetuated their own paternalistic attitudes about what is best for nursing and the public it serves. Medical statements on nursing still seem to relate more to the economic and social status of women than to actual needs of the public for nursing service.

Since the nursing profession has been an integral part of the American health and hospital system for over a century, the public has accepted much on the basis of faith that the highest caliber of nursing care possible was being made available to patients. In reality, this has not been the case. Moreover, public misconceptions have been fostered by the numerous and confusing levels of practice within nursing. In regard to employment practices, these levels may be used to the advantage or disadvantage of both patients and nurses. In few other professions are the well educated discriminated against as they are in nursing. In all other professions practitioners are evaluated on the basis of their educational qualifications and this should be the case with nursing. However, hospitals still prefer to employ the less well-educated woman to provide nursing services.

Given recent and current criticisms of poor quality in health care, the public would do well to turn more of its attention to developments in nursing and to the problems with which this group has to contend. For a century, defects in nursing service have provided an index to general defects in America's health care system. Patients have a right to have the best qualified nurses available to care for them when sick. Public evaluation and knowledge of the educational status and competence of nurses employed by any hospital is just as important as is the reputation of its medical staff. Many current criticisms of patient care can be traced to the inadequate employment of qualified nurses in health care settings.

The public can demand more of its nurses by utilizing them to a far greater extent than is done now. The nursing profession has made progress in improving the competence and expertise of its members and the public should capitalize on the improvements that can derive from having better prepared nurses. In the past, women in nursing have been forced into humble and virtuous servant roles in relation to the godlike role of the physician. Tied to the latter by public sanction and approval, nurses have too seldom questioned the human frailties of the physician. Nurses have always been able to observe errors in judgment committed by medical men but, not accorded professional status and credibility of judgment equal to these men, their criticisms have carried little weight with the public. More patient satisfaction could be obtained if nurses were utilized differently by patients and their families.

In their daily work nurses come into contact with almost every income group in society. They are strategically located in schools, industries, homes, hospitals, public health clinics, the military, and in all agencies caring for the sick. Their potential contributions can result in an improvement in health care if they, with the help of the public, would only develop it. It may be the best cure for what ails the American health care system.

Professional nursing must begin exerting open and public leadership in meeting consumer health needs. Dominant influences in health care will not yield to the private and quiet pleas of pacifying women: powerful, male-dominated groups, economically motivated, will not be reasonable with their interests and status threatened. Nurses must change their own attitudes toward themselves and their role. Narrow, single-minded educational and professional goals on the part of nursing leadership will not move nursing forward or improve health care. Their sense of responsibility and accountability must shift from that of meeting the needs of hospitals and physicians to meeting those of the patient and the public. The public can gain much by expanding its use of nurses and by supporting them in their efforts to exercise their potential in the area of health and hospital care.

In comparison with other occupational groups, nursing is very highly developed and more complex. Aides and practical nurses are accepted workers in nursing; educational programs for the various levels are well-defined. It is time nursing emerged to provide the care it can provide. Society can scarcely afford the waste caused by ineffective utilization of the talents and abilities of professionally and technically prepared nurses.

Healthy solutions to problems in health care require that the public become more accurately and fully informed about its health and hospital system to eliminate the mystery, myths, and confusion that surround the delivery of care. No small step in this direction is that of understanding the growth and development of American nursing since it has and does provide the largest number of practitioners in the health field.

Notes

CHAPTER I

1. Francis R. Packard, *Some Account of the Pennsylvania Hospital* (Philadelphia: Eagle Press, 1938), p. 2. (The title of this brief history is taken from an original publication of the same title written by Benjamin Franklin and published in 1754. The author of the 1938 version quoted extensively from Franklin's original work.)

2. N. I. Bowditch, *A History of the Massachusetts General Hospital* (Boston: John Wilson & Sons, 1851), p. 5.

3. John Fehrenbatch, "The Relation of Politics to the Hospital," *Transactions of the Fourth Annual Conference of the Association of Hospital Superintendents, 1902,* as reprinted in the *National Hospital Record,* Vol. II (December 1902), p. 37. (This association was renamed the American Hospital Association in 1908. Yearly transactions were published by different publishers throughout the country; hereafter they will be cited as *Transactions of the Association of Hospital Superintendents* or *A.H.A.,* with year and reference pages.)

4. Ibid., p. 36.

5. "Report of the Committee on How to Reduce the Annual Deficit," *Transactions of the Association of Hospital Superintendents, 1903,* p. 52.

6. "Editorial," *The Journal of the American Medical Association* Vol. 40 (January 31, 1903), p. 314 (hereafter cited as J.A.M.A.).

7. R. R. Ross, "Report of Committee on Hospital Progress," *Transactions of the A.H.A., 1909,* p. 412.

8. S. S. Goldwater, "The Appropriation of Public Funds for the Partial Support of Voluntary Hospitals in the United States and Canada," *Transactions of the A.H.A., 1909,* pp. 242-245.

9. Council on Medical Education and Hospitals of the American Medical Association, "Third Presentation of Hospital Data," *J.A.M.A.* Vol. 82 (January 1924), p. 118.

10. *Transactions of the Association of Hospital Superintendents,* *1905,* p. 56.

11. Charles Phillips Emerson, "The American Hospital Field," *Hospital Management,* Charlotte A. Aikens, ed. (Philadelphia: W. B. Saunders Company, 1911), p. 18.

12. Arthur Dean Bevan, "Medical Education in the United States: The Need of a Uniform Standard," *J.A.MA.* Vol. 51 (August 15, 1908), p. 566.

13. Abraham Flexner, "Hospitals, Medical Education and Research," *Transactions of the A.H.A., 1911,* pp. 368-369.

14. C. G. Parnall, "The Selection and Organization of Hospital Personnel," *Transactions of the A.H.A., 1920,* pp. 98-99.

15. *Transactions of the A.H.A., 1922,* p. 220.

16. William Allen Pusey, "Some Problems of Medicine," *J.A.M.A.* Vol. 82 (June 14, 1924), pp. 1905-1908.

17. David B. Skillman, "What Hospitals Can Do For and Against Socialized Medicine," *Transactions of the A.H.A., 1939,* p. 459.

18. Ibid., p. 460.

19. C. Rufus Rorem, *Capital Investment of Hospitals,* Publication No. 7 (Washington, D. C.: The Committee on the Costs of Medical Care, 1930), pp. 9-10.

20. Oscar R. Ewing, *The Nation's Health: A Report to the President* (Washington, D. C.: U. S. Government Printing Office, 1948), p. 10.

CHAPTER II

1. Mary Alice Snively, "A Uniform Curriculum for Training Schools," *Proceedings of the American Society of Superintendents of Training Schools for Nurses, 1895,* p. 26. (These proceedings were published by various publishers; only the name of the association, the year of the convention reports, and reference pages will be cited in subsequent notes.)

2. George H. M. Rowe, "Observations on Hospital Organization," *Transactions of the Association of Hospital Superintendents, 1902,* p. 65.

3. Ibid.

4. George P. Ludlam, "The Organization and Control of Training Schools," *New York Medical Journal,* Vol. 83 (April 1906), p. 851.

5. May Ayres Burgess, *Nurses, Patients, and Pocketbooks* (New York: Committee on the Grading of Nursing Schools, 1928), pp. 34-35.

6. Council on Medical Education and Hospitals of the American Medical Association, "Third Presentation of Hospital Data," *J.A.M.A.* Vol. 82 (January 1924), p. 118.

7. *Transactions of the Association of Hospital Superintendents, 1905,* pp. 56-58.

8. *Transactions of the Association of Hospital Superintendents, 1904,* pp. 170-172.

9. "Essentials of a Nursing Education," *National Hospital Record* Vol. XI (January 1908), pp. 2-3.

10. *Transactions of the A.H.A., 1908,* pp. 78-81.

11. "The Editorial Viewpoint," *National Hospital Record* Vol. XI (March 1908), p. 1.

12. *Proceedings of American Society of Superintendents of Training Schools, 1896,* p. 65.

13. G. W. Olson, "How the Small Hospital May Be Made Self-Supporting," *Transactions of the A.H.A., 1913,* p. 434.

14. Letter to the editor from R. L. Larsen, Chicago, Illinois, dated July 3, 1904, *New York Medical Journal* Vol. 80 (July 1904), p. 235.

15. Letter to the editor from Charles W. Kollock, dated July 16, 1904, *New York Medical Journal,* Vol. 80 (July 1904), p. 235.

16. Charlotte Mandeville Perry, "Pupil Nursing Outside the Hospital," *International Hospital Record,* Vol. 14 (October 1910), p. 23; also, "Pupil Nurses on Outside Cases," *International Hospital Record,* Vol. 17 (June 1914), p. 10. (Despite the title, this journal was strictly an American publication; formerly entitled the *National Hospital Record,* it was the official organ of the A.H.A. at the time of its inception.)

17. *Proceedings of the American Society of Superintendents of Training Schools, 1909,* pp. 186-187.

18. *Proceedings of the American Society of Superintendents of Training Schools, 1902,* pp. 30-33.

19. Ibid., p. 20.

20. Committee of Examiners of Registered Nurses, *Course of Study Recommended for the Training School for Nurses in Wisconsin* (Wisconsin: State Board of Health, 1913), p. 9.

21. See: *The Statutes of Ohio Regulating the Practice of Nursing and the Minimum Requirements for Recognized Training Schools* (Columbus, Ohio: The F. J. Heer Printing Company, 1915), p. 17; California State Board of Health, Bureau of Registration of Nurses, *Requirements and Course of Instruction for Accredited Schools of Nursing* (Sacramento: California State Printing Office, 1923), pp. 5, 7; Connecticut State Board of Examination and Registration of Nurses, *Survey of Train-*

ing Schools for Nurses (Connecticut: State Board of Examination and Registration of Nurses, 1916), pp. 4-5.

22. "Report on the Joint Session of the Council on Medical Education and Hospitals and the American Conference on Hospital Service," *J.A.M.A.* Vol. 100 (April 15, 1933), p. 1182.

23. Committee on the Grading of Nursing Schools, *Nursing Schools Today and Tomorrow* (New York: Privately published, 1934), pp. 159-160.

24. Robert E. Neff, "The Cost of Nursing Education to the Hospital," *American Journal of Nursing*, Vol. 29 (September 1929), p. 1119.

25. Ibid., p. 1120; also, for a very clear expression of this attitude, read Richard P. Borden, "Nursing Education from the Viewpoint of the Hospital Trustee," *Transactions of the A.H.A., 1925*, p. 119.

26. "Report of the Board of Trustees," *Transactions of the A.H.A., 1925*, p. 119.

27. Paul H. Douglas, *American Apprenticeship and Industrial Education* (New York: Privately published, 1921), pp. 20-21.

CHAPTER III

1. Mary Adelaide Nutting, "A Statistical Report of Working Hours in Training Schools," *Proceedings of the American Society of Superintendents of Training Schools, 1896*, p. 39.

2. Ibid., p. 36.

3. "The Eight-Hour Day," *National Hospital Record*, Vol. XI (January 15, 1908), p. 3.

4. Nutting to Meade, 6 December 1918, Nutting Papers, Archives of the Department of Nursing Education, Teachers College, Columbia University, New York, New York. (All subsequent letters cited are located in these Archives.)

5. Baker to Stewart, 20 June 1918.

6. Ibid.

7. Nutting to Baker, 29 June 1918.

8. W. A. Baker, "A Flagrant Injustice" (Typed manuscript, Nutting Papers), pp. 2-3.

9. Baker to Nutting, 12 July 1918.

10. Committee for the Study of Nursing Education, *Nursing and Nursing Education in the United States* (New York: The Macmillan Company, 1923), pp. 406-415.

11. *Proceedings of the National League of Nursing Education, 1915,* pp. 185-186 (hereafter cited as *N.L.N.E.*).

12. *Proceedings of the N.L.N.E., 1913,* p. 79.

13. Sacramento *Enquirer,* March 25, 1915.

14. Lila Pickhardt, "The Eight-Hour Law As Applied to Student Nurses," *Proceedings of the N.L.N.E., 1914,* pp. 109-110.

15. *Transactions of the A.H.A., 1915,* p. 130. (Material cited is an excerpt from the Court's decision.)

16. *Proceedings of the N.L.N.E., 1915,* pp. 184-185, 188.

17. "California's Eight-Hour Fight," *The Modern Hospital,* Vol. II (January 1914), p. 62.

18. "Editorial Comment," *American Journal of Nursing,* Vol. XIV (February 1914), pp. 332-333.

19. See the editorial comments in *The Nurse,* Vol. II (September 1921), pp. 5-6; also *The Nurse,* Vol. I (February 1921), p. 7. (The Chicago publishers of this periodical selected as their major focus the dispensing of propaganda against all legislative and regulatory measures designed to elevate standards in nursing education and practice. As a publication whose primary objective was to assist physicians in the organization and standardization of nursing, its content was of a political nature. See "Our Aims and Aspirations," *The Nurse,* Vol. I [August 16, 1920], p. 1.)

20. Jamme to Nutting, 1 May 1913.

21. Nutting to Jamme, 9 May 1913.

22. Nutting to Jamme, 3 May 1913.

23. Marie Hadden to Nutting, 11 October 1913.

24. *Transactions of the A.H.A., 1915,* p. 91.

25. *Proceedings of the N.L.N.E., 1915,* pp. 184-185.

26. Isabel M. Stewart, "Movement for Shorter Hours in Nurses' Training Schools," *American Journal of Nursing,* Vol. XIX (March 1919), pp. 439-440.

27. Ibid.

28. Committee for the Study of Nursing Education, *Nursing and Nursing Education in the United States,* p. 223.

CHAPTER IV

1. *Proceedings of the American Society of Superintendents of Training Schools, 1896,* p. 66.

2. Ibid., p. 67.

3. Ibid.

4. *Transactions of the A.H.A., 1913*, p. 277.

5. "Report on the Joint Session of the Council on Medical Education and the American Conference on Hospital Service," *J.A.M.A.*, Vol. 100 (April 15, 1933), p. 1179.

6. C. Rufus Rorem, "Comparative Costs of Undergraduate and Graduate Nursing," *J.A.M.A.*, Vol. 100 (April 15, 1933), p. 1180.

7. Committee on the Grading of Nursing Schools, *Nursing Schools Today and Tomorrow* (New York: Privately published, 1934), pp. 101-102.

8. Paul H. Fesler, "Hospital Nursing Costs: How Are They To Be Met?" *American Journal of Nursing*, Vol. 32 (June 1932), p. 638. (This paper was originally presented at a joint session [biennial convention] of the national nursing organizations held in San Antonio, Texas, April 2, 1932.)

9. C. W. Munger, "The School Committee and the Hospital Board," *Proceedings of the N.L.N.E., 1935*, pp. 134-136.

10. William O. Stillman, "A Successful Experiment in Educating Efficient Nurses for Persons of Moderate Income," *New York Medical Journal*, Vol. 91 (January 15, 1910), pp. 110-111.

11. John Dill Robertson, "Home and Public Health Nurses and Their Training," *J.A.M.A.*, Vol. 74 (January 14, 1920), pp. 481-483.

12. Ibid.

13. William James Mayo, "Observations on South America," *J.A.M.A.*, Vol. 75 (July 31, 1920), p. 314. (Although largely about nursing, the title of this article derives from the fact that Mayo had traveled in South America to observe systems of health care there.)

14. Richard Olding Beard, "The Trained Nurse of the Future," *J.A.M.A.*, Vol. 61 (December 13, 1913), p. 2151.

15. *Transactions of the A.H.A., 1913*, pp. 157-158. (Reference cited provides an interesting discussion of the problems created by correspondence courses.)

16. "Correspondence Schools for Nurses," *J.A.M.A.*, Vol. 60 (May 31, 1913), p. 1713; also, "The Doctor Again Picked Out For An Easy Mark," *J.A.M.A.*, Vol. 60 (February 20, 1913), p. 600; and, "Correspondence Nurses," *J.A.M.A.*, Vol. 88 (April 2, 1927), p. 1083. (Elaborate bulletins were prepared for correspondence courses; that of the Chautauqua School of Nursing, Jamestown, New York, dated 1933, provides a typical example. It is located along with various advertising materials in the Archives of the Department of Nursing Education, Teachers College, Columbia University.)

17. Chicago School of Nursing, *Splendid Opportunities* (Chicago: Chicago School of Nursing, 1932), p. 9. (This pamphlet is in the Nursing Archives, Teachers College, New York.)

18. *Transactions of the A.H.A., 1922*, p. 180.

19. Committee on the Grading of Nursing Schools, *Nursing Schools Today and Tomorrow*, p. 45.

20. Harlan Hoyt Horner, *Nursing Education and Practice in New York State with Suggested Remedial Measures* (Albany: The University of the State of New York Press, 1934), pp. 3-38.

21. Ibid., p. 7.

22. Ibid.

23. Elizabeth C. Burgess, "What Are Nurses Going to Do About It?" *Proceedings of the N.L.N.E., 1932*, pp. 49-50.

24. Ibid.

25. The economic status of nurses is reported on in the following articles by Lily Mary David published in *Monthly Labor Review*, Vol. 65: "The Economic Status of Nurses," (July 1947), pp. 20-27; "Working Conditions of Public-Health Nurses," (September 1947), pp. 302-303; "Working Conditions of Private Duty and Staff Nurses," (November 1947), pp. 544-548.

26. David, "The Economic Status of Nurses," p. 27.

27. Ibid., p. 21.

CHAPTER V

1. John Stuart Mill and Harriet Taylor Mill, *Essays on Sex Equality*, Alice S. Rossi, ed. (Chicago: University of Chicago Press, 1970), pp. 143-144.

2. Isabel M. Stewart, "Popular Fallacies About Nursing Education," Reprint from the *Modern Hospital*, Vol. XVII (November 1921), p. 2.

3. William Alexander Newman Dorland, *The Sphere of the Trained Nurse* (Address given at the Philadelphia School of Nursing, 27 May 1908).

4. Ibid.

5. "Nurses' Schools and Illegal Practice of Medicine," *J.A.M.A.*, Vol. 47 (December 1, 1906), p. 1835.

6. Edward J. Ill, "The Trained Nurse and the Doctor: Their Mutual Relation and Responsibilities," *The Journal of the Medical Society of New Jersey*, Vol. II (August 1905), pp. 36-38.

7. George P. Ludlam, "The Reaction in Training School Methods," *National Hospital Record,* Vol. XI (February 1908), p. 4.

8. Ibid.

9. William Alexander Newman Dorland, *The Autocracy of the Trained Nurse* (Philadelphia: Physicians' National Board of Regents, 1909), pp. 16-24.

10. Henry Beates, *The Status of Nurses: A Sociologic Problem* (Philadelphia: Physicians' National Board of Regents, 1909), p. 6.

11. Ibid., pp. 4-5.

12. Ibid., p. 17.

13. For expressions of concern over economic competition with nurses, see Theodore Potter, "The Nursing Problem," *New York Medical Journal,* Vol. 91 (May 1910), p. 998; "The Supply of Practical Nurses," *J.A.M.A.,* Vol. 72 (January 25, 1919), pp. 276-277; and "Medical News," *J.A.M.A.,* Vol. 95 (December 20, 1930), p. 1920.

14. Beates, *The Status of Nurses,* p. 21.

15. Ibid., p. 29.

16. W. Gilman Thompson, "The Relation of the Visiting and House Staff to the Care of Hospital Patients," *New York Medical Journal,* Vol. 83 (April 14, 1906), p. 744.

17. Theodore Potter, "The Nursing Problem," *New York Medical Journal,* Vol. 91 (May 1910), pp. 995-996.

18. For examples of these comments and others, see Thomas E. Satterthwaite, "Private Nurses and Nursing: With Recommendation for Their Betterment," *New York Medical Journal,* Vol. 91 (January 1910), pp. 108-110.

19. William Allen Pusey, "The Trend in Medical and Nursing Services," *J.A.M.A.,* Vol. 82 (June 14, 1924), p. 1916.

20. "Inaugural Address of the President of the American Medical Association," *J.A.M.A.,* Vol. 90 (June 16, 1928), p. 1920.

21. Winford H. Smith, "Again The Nursing Problem," *International Hospital Record,* Vol. 5 (May 1912), pp. 7-8.

22. "Report of the Council on Medical Education and Hospitals," *J.A.M.A.,* Vol. 84 (May 30, 1925), pp. 1655-1660.

23. "Minutes of the Seventy-Eighth Annual Session of the A.M.A.," *J.A.M.A.,* Vol. 88 (May 21, 1927), pp. 1642-1643. For more detailed information on committees on nursing appointed by the American Medical Association, see "Report of the Council on Medical Education and Hospitals," *J.A.M.A.,* Vol. 80 (June 30, 1923), pp. 1928-37; "Annual Congress on Medical Education, Medical Licensure, Public Health and Hospitals," *J.A.M.A.,* Vol. 80 (March 24, 1923), pp. 851-853; and "Report of

the Committee on Nurses and Nursing Education," *J.A.M.A.,* Vol. 88 (April 9, 1927), pp. 1175-80.

24. Richard Olding Beard, "Minority Report of Committee on Trained Nursing," *J.A.M.A.,* Vol. 80 (March 24, 1923), pp. 852-53.

25. *Transactions of the A.H.A., 1928,* pp. 288-289.

26. "Report on the Joint Session of the Council on Medical Education and Hospitals and the American Conference on Hospital Service," *J.A.M.A.,* Vol. 100 (April 15, 1933), p. 1170.

27. Ibid.

28. *Transactions of the A.H.A., 1928,* pp. 288-289.

29. *Proceedings of the N.L.N.E., 1935,* p. 258.

30. Ibid., p. 261.

31. Contents of report published in "Medical News," *J.A.MA.,* Vol. 91, (October 27, 1928), p. 1296.

32. *Transactions of the A.H.A., 1931,* p. 197.

Chapter VI

1. "Editorials," *J.A.M.A.,* Vol. 42 (June 4, 1904), p. 1499.

2. *Proceedings of the American Society of Superintendents of Training Schools, 1896,* p. 4.

3. Ibid.

4. Ibid., pp. 4-6.

5. Lavinia L. Dock, *A History of Nursing,* Vol. III (New York: G. P. Putnam's Sons, 1912), p. 117.

6. *Proceedings of the American Society of Superintendents of Training Schools, 1897,* p. 5.

7. Ibid.

8. *Proceedings of the American Society of Superintendents of Training Schools, 1895,* pp. 45-46.

9. *Proceedings of the American Society of Superintendents of Training Schools, 1897,* p. 5.

10. George H. M. Rowe, "Observations on Hospital Organization," *Transactions of the Association of Hospital Superintendents, 1902* (in *National Hospital Record*), p. 64.

11. Ibid.

12. Lavinia L. Dock, "The Duty of This Society in Public Work," *Proceedings of the American Society of Superintendents of Training Schools, 1903,* p. 77.

13. Ibid., pp. 77-78.

14. Ibid., pp. 78-79.

15. Nurses were quite divided on the issue and problem of superintendents cooperating with the hospital association. For a discussion indicating this divisiveness, see *Proceedings of the American Society of Superintendents of Training Schools, 1909,* pp. 20-26, 93-94. (For a recording of decision to admit superintendents as members of the A.H.A., see *Transactions of the A.H.A., 1913,* p. 91. Other members of the hospital staff, such as surgeons, were also admitted to membership.)

16. Luella L. Goold, "Suggestions As To Possibilities of Student Government in Hospital Training Schools," *Proceedings of the American Society of Superintendents of Training Schools, 1910,* p. 135. (Her comments are directed toward student discipline which applied equally to adult women [the superintendents] in the hospital system.)

17. Ibid., p. 130.

18. Thomas E. Satterthwaite, "Private Nurses and Nursing: With Recommendation for Their Betterment," *New York Medical Journal,* Vol. 91 (January 15, 1910), p. 110.

19. Ibid., pp. 109-110.

20. *Proceedings of the American Society of Superintendents of Training Schools, 1911,* p. 19.

21. Ibid., p. 20.

22. *Proceedings of the American Society of Superintendents of Training Schools, 1912,* pp. 126-133.

23. Ibid., p. 133.

24. Isabel M. Stewart, "Notes on the Founding of Nursing Departments" (Unpublished typewritten manuscript, dated 1918, Nursing Archives, Teachers College, New York), pp. 4-5.

25. *Transactions of the A.H.A., 1908,* p. 207.

26. Ella Phillips Crandall, "Report of Committee on the Training of Nurses," *Transactions of the A.H.A., 1916,* p. 47.

27. *Committee on Training of Nurses of the Hospital Conference of the City of New York* (copy of resolution adopted February 13, 1912) Nursing Archives, Teachers College, New York, p. 1.

28. Crandall, *Transactions of the A.H.A., 1916,* p. 49.

29. Mary Jean Hurdley, "How Can Training Schools Best Co-Operate With Educational Institutions," *Proceedings of the American Society of Superintendents of Training Schools, 1912,* p. 26.

30. Ibid., p. 27.

31. John Stuart Mill and Harriet Taylor Mill, *Essays on Sex Equality,* Alice S. Rossi, ed. (Chicago: The University of Chicago Press, 1970), p. 130.

32. "The Supply of Practical Nurses," *J.A.M.A.*, Vol. 72 (January 25, 1919), pp. 276-277; also, in this Journal, "The Nursing Problem," Vol. 75 (July 31, 1920), p. 324. (The following periodical published by physicians dispensed propaganda against legislation and the elevation of standards throughout the 1920's: *The Nurse,* Vol. I [August 1920], p. 1; and Vol. II [September 1921], pp. 5-6.)

33. Richard P. Borden, "Nursing Education from the Viewpoint of the Hospital Trustees," *Transactions of the A.H.A., 1929*, p. 277.

34. *Proceedings of the N.L.N.E., 1936*, p. 267.

35. "Minutes, Annual Session of House of Delegates of American Medical Association," *J.A.M.A.*, Vol. 129 (December 22, 1945), p. 1191.

CHAPTER VII

1. Rozella M. Schlotfeldt, "Nursing Is Health Care," *Nursing Outlook,* Vol. 20 (April 1972), p. 245.

2. American Nurses Association, *A Position Paper* (New York: American Nurses Association, 1965).

3. John H. Knowles, "Medical School, Teaching Hospital, and Social Responsibility," *Teaching Hospitals,* John H. Knowles, ed. (Cambridge, Massachusetts: Harvard University Press, 1966), p. 126.

4. A.M.A. Committee on Nursing, "Medicine and Nursing in the 1970's: A Position Statement," *J.A.M.A.*, Vol. 213 (September 14, 1970), pp. 1881-1883.

5. Raymond S. Duff and August B. Hollinghead, *Sickness and Society* (New York: Harper & Row, Publishers, 1968), p. 373.

Bibliography

THE MOST VALUABLE primary and secondary sources for this research were archival materials from collections on nursing, medicine, and hospitals. Those used for this study were the Archives of the Department of Nursing Education and the Nutting Collection, both at Teachers College, Columbia University in New York; the Annie W. Goodrich Papers of the Collection of Historical Materials, Yale University School of Nursing in New Haven; and the New York Academy of Medicine Library in New York City.

The most important material on the policies and practices influencing twentieth-century developments in the health care system is found in official documents: specifically official studies and proceedings of the two original nursing organizations and their successor groups, and those of organized medicine and hospital administration. An examination of yearly proceedings of the American Nurses' Association, the National League of Nursing, the American Medical Association, and the American Hospital Association provided excellent detailed indicators of the prevailing attitudes and institutional procedures guiding the growth of nursing, medicine, and hospitals.

Unfortunately, most current feminist writings neither recognize nor comment on the problems of women who work in the health field other than those who are physicians. Germaine Greer in *The Female Eunuch* is the only current feminist author who makes any mention of nurses and their difficulties in caring for the sick.

DOCUMENTARY MATERIALS

American Hospital Association. *Transactions of Annual Conference,* 1908-1950.

American Medical Association. Various minutes, annual proceedings, and reports of committees. *The Proceedings and Journal of the American Medical Association,* 1893-1950.

American Nurses' Association. *Annual Proceedings and Journal of the American Nurses' Association,* 1900-1950.

————. *A Position Paper.* New York: American Nurses' Association, 1967.

————. *Facts About Nursing.* A Statistical Report. New York: American Nurses' Association, 1967.

————. *Facts About Nursing: A Statistical Summary, 1970-71 Edition.* New York: American Nurses' Association, 1972.

American Society of Superintendents of Training Schools for Nurses. *Proceedings of Annual Conventions,* 1894-1912.

Association of Hospital Superintendents of the United States and Canada. *Transactions of Annual Conferences,* 1900-1907.

Board of Education. *Nursing Education in Minnesota.* A Report Authorized by the Board of Education of the State of Minnesota. Edited by Louise Muller. St. Paul, Minnesota: Department of Education, 1937.

Burgess, May Ayres. *Nurses, Patients, and Pocketbooks.* Report of a Study of the Economics of Nursing. New York: Committee on the Grading of Nursing Schools, 1928.

Committee on the Grading of Nursing Schools. *Nursing Schools Today and Tomorrow.* A Report of the Committee on the Grading of Nursing Schools. New York: By the Committee, 1934.

The Committee on the Costs of Medical Care. *Medical Care for the American People.* The Final Report of the Committee on the Costs of Medical Care. Chicago: The University of Chicago Press, 1932.

Connecticut Training School for Nurses. *Annual Reports.* 1873-1900.

Curran, Jean A., and Bunge, Helen L. *Better Nursing: A Study of Nursing Care and Education in Washington.* A Report of the University of Washington Advisory Committee on Nursing Service and Training Programs of the State of Washington. Seattle: University of Washington Press, 1951.

Ewing, Oscar R. *The Nation's Health: A Report to the President.* Washington, D. C.: U. S. Government Printing Office, 1948.

Horner, Harlan Hoyt. *Nursing Education and Practice in New York State With Suggested Remedial Measures.* Albany: The University of the State of New York Press, 1934.

Johns, Ethel, and Pfefferkorn, Blanche. *An Activity Analysis of Nursing.* A Report of the Committee on the Grading of Nursing Schools. New York, 1934.

National League of Nursing Education. *Proceedings of Annual Conventions.* 1912-1950.

————. *Standard Curriculum for Schools of Nursing.* A Report Prepared by the Committee on Education. Baltimore: Waverly Press, 1917.

————. *A Curriculum Guide for Schools of Nursing.* New York: National League of Nursing Education, 1937.

Nutting, Mary Adelaide. *Educational Status of Nursing.* U. S. Bureau of Education, Bulletin 7, No. 475. Washington: U. S. Government Printing Office, 1912.

Park, Clyde W. *The Cooperative System of Education.* U. S. Bureau of Education, Bulletin No. 2. Washington, D. C.: U. S. Government Printing Office, 1916.

President's Commission on the Health Needs of the Nation. *Building America's Health: A Report to the President.* Vol. I. Washington, D. C.: U. S. Government Printing Office, 1953.

President's Commission on the Health Needs of the Nation. *Building America's Health: America's Health Status, Needs and Resources.* Vol. 2. A Report to the President. Washington, D. C.: U. S. Government Printing Office, 1953.

President's Commission on the Health Needs of the Nation. *Building America's Health: Financing A Health Program for America.* Vol. 4. A Report to the President. Washington, D. C.: U. S. Government Printing Office, 1953.

Rorem, C. Rufus. *Capital Investment in Hospitals.* Publication No. 7. Washington, D. C.: The Committee on the Costs of Medical Care, 1930.

Stewart, Isabel M. *Developments in Nursing Education Since 1918.* Department of the Interior, Bureau of Education. Bulletin No. 20. Washington, D. C.: U. S. Government Printing Office, 1921.

MONOGRAPHS AND GENERAL BOOKS

Abdellah, Faye G., and Levine, Eugene. *Better Patient Care Through Nursing Research.* New York: The Macmillan Company, 1965.

Aikens, Charlotte A. (ed.). *Hospital Management.* Philadelphia: W. B. Saunders Company, 1911.

Batey, Marjorie V. (ed.). *Communicating Nursing Research: Methodological Issues.* Boulder, Colorado: Western Interstate Commission for Higher Education, 1970.

Bowditch, N. I. *A History of the Massachusetts General Hospital.* Boston. John Wilson & Sons, 1851.

Bridgman, Margaret. *Collegiate Education for Nursing.* New York: Russell Sage Foundation, 1953.

Brown, Esther Lucile. *Nursing for the Future.* New York: Russell Sage Foundation, 1948.

Burling, Temple; Lentz, Edith M.; and Wilson, Robert N. *The Give and Take In Hospitals: A Study of Human Organization In Hospitals.* New York: G. P. Putnam's Sons, 1956.

Committee on the Study of Nursing Education. *Nursing and Nursing Education in the United States.* New York: The Macmillan Company, 1923.

Committee on the Function of Nursing. *A Program for the Nursing Profession.* New York: The Macmillan Company, 1948.

Communicating Nursing Research. Edited by Marjorie V. Batey. (Research Conference held at Salt Lake City, Utah, April 29-May 1, 1970. Supported by Research Grant NU002890-03, Division of Nursing, National Institutes of Health.) Boulder, Colorado: Western Interstate Commission for Higher Education, 1970.

Cook, Sir Edward. *The Life of Florence Nightingale.* New York: The Macmillan Company, 1942.

Cray, Ed. *In Failing Health: The Medical Crisis and the A. M. A.* New York: The Bobbs-Merrill Company, Inc., 1970.

Cremin, Lawrence A. *The Transformation of the School.* New York: Alfred A. Knopf, Inc., 1961.

Curti, Merle. *The Social Ideas of American Educators.* Paperback ed. revised. Totowa, New Jersey: Littlefield, Adams & Company, 1966. (First published in 1934; New York: Charles Scribner's Sons.)

Davis, Fred (ed.). *The Nursing Profession: Five Sociological Essays.* New York: John Wiley and Sons, Inc., 1966.

Dewey, John. *Democracy and Education.* New York: The Macmillan Company, 1916.

Douglas, Paul H. *American Apprenticeship and Industrial Education.* New York: Privately published, 1921.

Duff, Raymond S., and Hollingshead, August B. *Sickness and Society.* New York: Harper & Row, Publishers, 1968.

Ehrenreich, Barbara, and Ehrenreich, John. *The American Health Empire: Power, Profits, and Politics.* New York: Vintage Books, 1971.

Epstein, Cynthia Fuchs, and Goode, William J. *The Other Half: Roads To Women's Equality.* Englewood Cliffs, New Jersey: Prentice-Hall, Inc. 1971.

Freidson, Eliot (ed.). *The Hospital In Modern Society.* New York: The Free Press of Glencoe, 1963.

Galbraith, John Kenneth. *The New Industrial State.* Paperback ed. New York: The New American Library, Inc., 1968.

Gelinas, Agnes. *Nursing and Nursing Education.* New York: The Commonwealth Fund, 1946.

Georgopoulos, Basil S., and Mann, Floyd C. *The Community General Hospital.* New York: The Macmillan Company, 1962.

Greer, Germaine. *The Female Eunuch.* New York: Bantam Books, Inc., 1972. (First published in 1971; New York: McGraw-Hill Book Company.)

Hoyt, Edwin P. *Your Health Insurance: A Story of Failure.* New York: The John Day Company, 1970.

Janeway, Elizabeth. *Man's World, Woman's Place: A Study In Social Mythology.* New York: William Morrow and Company, Inc., 1971.

King, Imogene M. *Toward a Theory for Nursing.* New York: John Wiley and Sons, Inc., 1971.

Knowles, John H. (ed.). *The Teaching Hospital.* Cambridge, Massachusetts: Harvard University Press, 1966.

Lambertsen, Eleanor C. *Education for Nursing Leadership.* Philadelphia: J. B. Lippincott Company, 1958.

Lapp, John A., and Ketcham, Dorothy. *Hospital Law.* Milwaukee, Wisconsin: The Bruce Publishing Company, 1926.

Lesnik, Milton J., and Anderson, Bernice E. *Nursing Practice and the Law.* 2d ed. revised. Philadelphia: J. B. Lippincott Company, 1962. (First published in 1947 under the title *Legal Aspects of Nursing.* Philadelphia: J. B. Lippincott Company.)

MacDonald, Gwendoline. *Development of Standards and Accreditation*

In Collegiate Nursing Education. New York: Teachers College Press, 1965.

Mill, John Stuart, and Mill, Harriet Taylor. *Essays on Sex Equality.* Edited by Alice S. Rossi. Chicago: The University of Chicago Press, 1970.

Montag, Mildred L. *The Education of Nursing Technicians.* Paperback ed. New York: John Wiley and Sons, Inc., 1971. (First published in 1951; New York: G. P. Putnam's Sons.)

Morgan, Robin (ed.). *Sisterhood Is Powerful: An Anthology of Writing From the Women's Liberation Movement.* New York: Vintage Books, 1970.

Norris, Catherine M. (ed.). *Proceedings of The Second Nursing Theory Conference.* Topeka, Kansas: Robert R. Sanders, 1970.

―――――. *Proceedings of The Third Nursing Theory Conference.* Topeka, Kansas: Robert R. Sanders, 1970.

Nutting, Mary Adelaide. *A Sound Economic Basis for Schools of Nursing.* New York: G. P. Putnam's Sons, 1926.

Packard, Francis R. *Some Account of the Pennsylvania Hospital.* Philadelphia: Engle Press, 1938.

Park, Clyde W. *The Co-Operative System of Education.* A Reprint of Bulletin No. 37. Series of 1916 With Additions. U. S. Bureau of Education. Cincinnati, Ohio: University of Cincinnati, 1925.

Pirenne, Henri. *Economic and Social History of Medieval Europe.* New York: Harcourt, Brace, Inc., 1937.

Roberts, Mary M. *American Nursing: History and Interpretation.* New York: The Macmillan Company, 1955. (First printed in 1954; New York: The Macmillan Company.)

Scrimshaw, Stewart. *Apprenticeship.* New York: McGraw-Hill Book Company, Inc., 1932.

Shryock, Richard Harrison. *The Development of Modern Medicine.* Philadelphia: University of Pennsylvania Press, 1936.

Stewart, Isabel M., and Austin, Anne L. *A History of Nursing.* 5th ed. revised. New York: G. P. Putnam's Sons, 1962.

Taylor, Carol. *In Horizontal Orbit: Hospitals and the Cult of Efficiency.* New York: Holt, Rinehart and Winston, 1970.

Woody, Thomas. *A History of Women's Education in the United States.* Vol. II. New York: The Science Press, 1929.

PAMPHLETS AND NEWSPAPERS

Ballard School. *Practical Nurse Training.* New York: Young Women's Christian Association, 1940-1941.

Beates, Henry. *The Status of Nurses: A Sociologic Problem.* Philadelphia: Physicians' National Board of Regents, 1909.

Bulletin of The Chautauqua School of Nursing, Jamestown, New York, 1933.

California State Department of Public Health, Bureau of Registration of Nurses. *Requirements and Course of Instruction for Accredited Schools of Nursing.* Sacramento: California State Printing Office, 1931.

California State Board of Health, Bureau of Registration of Nurses. *Requirements and Course of Instruction for Accredited Schools of Nursing.* Sacramento: California State Printing Office, 1923.

Chicago School of Nursing. *Amazing Opportunities In Nursing for the Ambitious Woman.* Chicago: Chicago School of Nursing, 1926.

————. *Splendid Opportunities.* Chicago: Chicago School of Nursing, 1932, 1942.

Committee of Examiners of Registered Nurses. *Course of Study Recommended for the Training School for Nurses in Wisconsin.* Wisconsin: State Board of Health, 1913.

Connecticut State Board of Examination and Registration of Nurses. *Survey of Training Schools for Nurses.* Connecticut: Issued by State Board of Examination and Registration of Nurses, 1916.

Dorland, William Alexander Newman. *The Sphere of the Trained Nurse.* Philadelphia: Philadelphia School of Nursing, 1908.

————. *The Autocracy of the Trained Nurse.* Philadelphia: Physicians' National Board of Regents, 1909.

The Statutes of Ohio Regulating the Practice of Nursing and the Minimum Requirements for Recognized Training Schools. Columbus, Ohio: The F. J. Heer Printing Company, 1915.

Index

About the Author

Jo Ann Ashley, a graduate of a hospital school of nursing, has a doctorate from Teachers College, Columbia University. She taught at the City College of New York, Pennsylvania State University, and Northern Illinois University before joining the School of Nursing at Texas Woman's University. She has served on the board of trustees for the Nurses Coalition for Action in Politics of the American Nurses' Association and is an active speaker and writer on aspects of the nursing profession.

Other Teachers College Press Publications on Nursing

PRESENT REALITIES/FUTURE IMPERATIVES IN
    NURSING EDUCATION: PAPERS FROM THE 12TH
    ANNUAL STEWART CONFERENCE ON RESEARCH
    IN NURSING

Louise Fitzpatrick, Editor

THE NURSING PROCESS: PROCEEDINGS OF THE
    10TH ANNUAL STEWART CONFERENCE ON
    RESEARCH IN NURSING

Marie M. Seedor, Editor

EVALUATION OF GRADUATES OF ASSOCIATE DEGREE
    NURSING PROGRAMS

Mildred E. Montag

LEARNING NEEDS OF REGISTERED NURSES

Elmina M. Price

NURSING LEADERSHIP BEHAVIOR IN GENERAL
    HOSPITALS

Elizabeth Hagen and Luverne Wolff